# A Clinician's Guide to Nutrition in HIV and AIDS

Cade Fields-Gardner, MS, RD

Cynthia A. Thomson, MS, RD

Sara S. Rhodes, RD

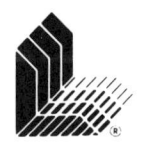

THE AMERICAN DIETETIC ASSOCIATION

**Library of Congress Cataloging-in-Publication Data**

Fields-Gardner, Cade.
 A clinician's guide to nutrition in HIV and AIDS / Cade Fields-Gardner, Cynthia A. Thomson, Sara S. Rhodes.
    p. cm.
 Includes bibliographical references and index.
 ISBN 0-88091-148-4
 1. AIDS (Disease)—Diet therapy.  I. Thomson, Cynthia.  II. Rhodes, Sara.  III. Title.
 [DNLM: 1. Acquired Immunodeficiency Syndrome—diet therapy.  2. Nutrition.  3. HIV Infections—diet therapy.  WC 530.2 F461c 1997]
 RC607.A26F54  1997
 616.97'920654—dc20
 DNLM/DLC
 for Library of Congress                                                96-36494
                                                                          CIP

© 1997, The American Dietetic Association. All rights reserved. No part of this publication may be reproduced, stored in a retrieval system, or transmitted in any form or by any means, without the prior written consent of the publisher. Printed in the United States of America.

The views expressed in this publication are those of the authors and do not necessarily reflect policies and/or official positions of The American Dietetic Association. Mention of product names in this publication does not constitute endorsement by the authors or The American Dietetic Association. The American Dietetic Association disclaims responsibility for the application of the information contained herein.

10  9  8  7  6  5  4  3  2  1

# Preface

This book is long overdue and yet is probably being published prematurely. Vital new information about the role of nutrition in the human immunodeficiency virus (HIV) and the acquired immunodeficiency syndrome (AIDS) is being collected in studies and by clinical experience on a daily basis.

It has been well established that nutrition and its supporting therapies are as essential to the overall treatment plan for HIV disease as is any other component. Nutrition should be seen as an integrated medical and psychosocial therapy. If any medication showed as much promise as nutrition interventions, conferences would be filled with eager clinicians and their patients.

New combinations of antiretroviral therapies and a global vaccination initiative have given scientists and clinicians hope for a cure for HIV infection and disease. It has been suggested that by reducing the impact of HIV viral replication on immune function, many of the detrimental conditions associated with HIV disease would be ameliorated. However, based on preliminary data from the XI International Conference on AIDS (1996) and more complete data reported at the International Nutrition and HIV Conference (1997), malnutrition that occurs in HIV disease may not be reversed by antiretroviral agents. In other words, once malnutrition is associated with HIV disease, it becomes an independent disease state that requires nutrition-related strategies for appropriate management.

There is a tremendous interest in nutrition-related interventions of HIV disease for many reasons. From the client's or patient's perspective, nutrition therapies are often a part of the medical plan over which they have control. From the clinician's perspective, nutrition may range from an exciting primary or prophylactic therapy to the nuisance that one must deal with as an adjunct to other medical therapies. To many, nutrition denotes a more glamorous and magical medical therapy. Discussion has surrounded both general and detailed questions of nutrient provision and preservation of nutritional status. Recently, groups such as the National HIV Nutrition Team and a dietetic practice group of The American Dietetic Association have formed to specifically address these issues across the boundaries of clinical, community, foodservice, and psychosocial-economic interests.

The successful use of medications requires compliance. However, nutrition interventions, particularly those aimed at prevention, demand commitment. The commitment required by both clients and clinicians is to individualize and integrate these therapies. Dietitians must continue to monitor and adjust their nutritional recommendations. An overall perspective allows us to keep in mind our goal to preserve and strengthen the whole person while we strive to address seemingly single problems. Individuals with hands-on experience in integrating nutrition-related interventions now see the need for this paradigm shift to serve our clients more appropriately and more successfully. As one of our greatest challenges, successful completion of this comprehensive task will allow us the opportunity to use every aspect of our training as clinicians and all our compassion as human beings.

We would like to thank the following reviewers for their valuable contributions:

*Reviewers in HIV/AIDS DPG*
Marcy Fenton, MS, RD
Coordinator for DPG Reviewers
Chair, HIV/AIDS DPG
HIV Nutrition Advocate, AIDS Project Los Angeles
Los Angeles, California

Satindar Dua, MS, RD
Nutrition Consultant
Los Angeles, California

Amber Ellis, RD
Training/Implementation Consultant
Computrition
Chatsworth, California
(formerly with AIDS Healthcare Foundation
Los Angeles, California)

Renee Hoffinger, MHSE, RD
Nutrition Commentator & Consultant
Gainesville, Florida

Jennifer Jensen, MS, MBA, RD
Nutrition Power
Santa Monica, California

Janelle L'Heureux, RD
Nutrition & HIV Program Volunteer
AIDS Project Los Angeles
Los Angeles, California

Anita Patil, MS, RD
Director of Nutritional Services
Country Villa South Nursing Center
Los Angeles, California

Stephanie Larmour Sanders, MS, RD
Metabolic Support Team
Cedars-Sinai Medical Center
Los Angeles, California

Ellyn C. Silverman, MPH, RD
ECS Nutrition Services
Long Beach, California

Greg Wine, RD
St. John's Hospital
Santa Monica, California

*Additional Reviewers*
Amy E. Inman-Felton, RD
Quality Nutrition Services
Wheaton, Illinois
(formerly Nutrition Support Dietitian
Edward Hines VA Hospital
Maywood, Illinois)

Donna Pertel, MEd, RD
Health Care Financing Team
American Dietetic Association
Chicago, Illinois
(formerly Clinical Dietitian
Northwestern Memorial Hospital
Chicago, Illinois)

Chris Rosenbloom, PhD, RD
Associate Professor
Department of Nutrition
Georgia State University
Atlanta, Georgia

We would particularly like to acknowledge the many contributions of Carol Capozza, RD, Advanced Infusion Services, Case Management Service, Emeryville, California.

We hope that you will find this guide a valuable resource and a foundation on which to build your commitment to working with patients and colleagues to make HIV and AIDS truly manageable. Our goal is to assure our patients' hopes and expectations for a full and satisfying life.

Cade Fields-Gardner

# Contents

Preface   iii

## 1 Overview and Nutritional Implications in HIV and AIDS   1
History of AIDS   2
Definitions of HIV and AIDS   3
Pathophysiological Process of HIV Infection   6
Laboratory Indicators of HIV Infection   7
Modes of Transmission   8
Epidemiology   8
Clinical Manifestations of HIV Disease   9
Nutritional Implications of AIDS   13
Summary   15

## 2 Nutrition Screening and Assessment   18
Nutrition Screening   18
Stages of HIV Infection   21
Medical Nutrition Therapy Protocols   22
Nutrition Assessment   24
Review of Medical and Social History   37
Importance of Exercise   37
Measuring Outcomes of Medical Nutrition Therapy   40
Summary   40

## 3 Oral Nutrition Interventions   43
Guidelines for Healthy Eating   44
Common Dietary Problems   48
Vitamin and Mineral Supplementation   53
Oral Nutrition Supplements   54
Alternative Therapies   56
Nutrition Counseling Skills   57
Nutritional Needs of HIV-Infected Women During Pregnancy and Lactation   58
Summary   61

## 4 Enteral and Parenteral Nutrition Strategies   65
Goals for Nutrition Support   65
Nutrition Assessment   67
Individualized Nutrition Support   67
Enteral Feeding   73
Parenteral Support   80
Role of the Registered Dietitian   89
Summary   91

## 5 Assessment and Intervention Issues in Various Health Care Settings   93
Inpatient Setting   93
Outpatient and Clinic Settings   97
Home Health Care Settings   99
Use of Health Services by Persons with HIV Disease   104
Managed Care   105
Community-Based Nutriiton Programs in AIDS Care   106
Hospice Setting   109
HIV/AIDS Medical Nutrition Therapy Protocol   110
Summary   111

## Appendixes

## A Glossary of HIV/AIDS Terminology   113

## B Nutrition Assessment   120
HIV/AIDS Medical Nutrition Therapy Protocol   121
Walter Reed Staging Classification for HIV Infection   136
Karnofsy Scale of Performance Status   136
Standardized Methods for Measuring Height and Weight   137
Body Mass Index Values   137
Anthropometric Values and Procedures   138
Bioelectrical Impedance Analysis Protocol and Report   142
Methods for Measuring Hand Dynamometry   145

## C Selected In-service Outlines   146

## D Resources   166
Food Programs Serving Meals to Clients with HIV/AIDS   166
Commercial Products   169
Professional Resources   170
Buyer's Clubs   173
Current Clinical Trials   173
Suggested Resources for HIV Case Managers   174

Index   175

# 1
# Overview and Nutritional Implications in HIV and AIDS

The human immunodeficiency virus (HIV) is one of the major human and scientific challenges of the 20th century. It is likely that no other infectious epidemic in our lifetime has created as much fear as HIV infection and thus moved scientists and journalists alike to hyperbole. Consequently, in a recent poll (1), 90% of those sampled in the United States concurred that acquired immunodeficiency syndrome (AIDS), the condition to which HIV infection may progress, is a source of worry for everyone, not just homosexual men and intravenous drug users, still the two groups at highest risk for the disease. This is true even though some people who are concerned about contracting the disease may be at very limited risk for infection.

Comparisons with other widespread diseases can be illuminating. The bubonic plague killed more people proportionately than any other disease in history. Starting in 1320, the plague reduced China's population from 125 million to 90 million (2). During the following decades, tens of millions of people were killed by the plague (caused by *Yersinia pestis*), including some 25 million Europeans.

Two centuries later, smallpox wiped out entire populations in the New World. Smallpox killed half the population in Mexico in 1520 and led to a civil war in Peru after killing the emperor in 1526 (3). More recently, in 1918, influenza claimed more victims than the first World War; 2 million people died of the flu.

Although HIV has not wiped out entire populations or started a war, the number of persons affected is still significant. Worldwide, the cumulative number of deaths due to HIV and AIDS as of December 1996 was 6.4 million (4). More than 1.5 million Americans are estimated to have been infected with HIV. Developing countries, especially in Africa, have the greatest number of cases. In sub-Saharan Africa, 14 million people are estimated to have HIV infection (4).

Although some analysts perhaps have overdramatized the impact of HIV disease, optimists proclaim that the war is almost over, thanks to a new class of antiretroviral drugs known as protease inhibitors and combination therapies, along with improved therapies against AIDS-defining infections (5). People with HIV are living longer due largely to better treatment, but this improvement is occurring primarily in more affluent countries such as the United States, Canada, some European nations, and Australia. In these countries, people with HIV can receive advanced high-tech medical care and access to costly protease inhibitors. This does not mean that all infected persons who live in these countries can afford the new therapies and drugs. Some persons infected with HIV are poor, homeless, and uninsured. Dependence on public assistance programs can be competitive and tenuous.

Much has been learned about HIV disease in the last 15 years, and efforts are aimed at transforming it from a fatal disease to a chronic condition. Today many people with HIV survive longer and experience an improved quality of life. The long-term effects of the new HIV therapies are often unknown, and patient responses vary. Some patients develop resistance over time to their antiretroviral "cocktails" or experience intolerable adverse reactions to the drugs.

The virus that causes AIDS is resilient and has outwitted strategies of scientists and clinicians in the past. HIV can be in tissues that are difficult to assess or screen and thus may escape detection. It can also survive by mutating into different strains, as do other infectious agents. This has reduced the efficacy of new antiviral drugs in the past. The virus can reproduce itself so rapidly (potentially two to three generations in 1 or 2 hours) that mutations are quick and can easily overcome drug therapies if an effective drug level is not maintained (6).

Unless a vaccine or a cure is found, the challenge remains for health care providers specializing in HIV, including dietitians, to continue supporting efforts to prevent the spread of this virus and to do their best in managing HIV disease. Improved quality of life is the ultimate goal for the patient.

## History of AIDS

It is speculated that in the late 1970s and early 1980s HIV infection spread among heterosexuals in east and central Africa and primarily among homosexual and bisexual males in the Americas, western Europe, Australia, and New Zealand (7). In 1981 AIDS was first recognized in the United States as an immune disorder in five homosexual men who presented with *Pneumocystis carinii* pneumonia (PCP). On investigation, it was suggested that the unknown cause of this immunodeficiency could be transmitted through sexual contact.

The acquired immunodeficiency syndrome was diagnosed in a person with hemophilia in 1983 for the first time and traced to a blood transfusion. That same year the cause of AIDS was identified as HIV and was determined to be carried in bodily fluids. During this time, levels of CD4 cells, T cells that orchestrate the function of the immune system, were used to determine the relative degree of immune destruction. Additionally, the measurement of CD4 levels was instituted as a means to monitor the potential for opportunistic events such as PCP or Kaposi's sarcoma.

Also in 1983, Luc Montagnier with the Pasteur Institute in Paris and Robert Gallo with the National Institutes of Health in the United States issued separate reports (7, 8) that each group had isolated HIV about the same time in their separate laboratories. That same year, reports increased of HIV transmission in US heterosexuals and women.

In 1985 Montagnier and Gallo independently reported the genetic sequence of HIV. Also that year, a second variant of HIV (HIV-2) was identified. A third development in 1985, which would help slow the spread of HIV, was the introduction of an HIV antibody test to screen the US blood supply.

In 1987 the first AIDS drug, the antiretroviral agent azidothymidine (AZT), now known as zidovudine, was approved for use for HIV infection. Community AIDS activists and health care providers advocated for parallel track testing of new therapies (providing ongoing investigation while the drug is made available for patient use) and a streamlined approval process by the US Food and Drug Administration (FDA). Other antiretroviral agents were introduced, along with improved preventive treatments for opportunistic infections. In 1995 the first protease inhibitor, saquinavir mesylate (Invirase, Roche Laboratories, Nutley, NJ 07110), became commercially available. In 1996 two other protease inhibitors, ritonavir (Norvir, Abbott Laboratories, Abbott Park, IL 60064) and indinavir sulfate (Crixivan, Merck & Co, West Point, PA 19486), were approved by the FDA. A report presented at the XIth International Conference of AIDS in Vancouver in 1996 suggested that a new multidrug regimen could reduce the viral burden (the level of virus in the blood). Viral load testing was added to the laboratory evaluations to determine the efficacy of antiretroviral therapy and to predict the potential rate of disease progression and survival.

With these new drugs, some HIV-infected persons were beginning to live longer and show an improvement in symptoms. For the first time in years, the survival rates in the United States began to improve. *Science* hailed the pharmaceutical advance against HIV as the number one breakthrough of the year (9). When 1996 ended, potent new drugs and new research about chemokines (a hormonelike protein that is released by certain cells to regulate immune cell activity) were proclaimed as holding great promise in the battle against AIDS.

The year 1997 brought an additional protease inhibitor, nelfinavir mesylate (Viracept, Agouron Pharmaceuticals, La Jolla, CA 92037), to the market. Additionally, further progress was made in prophylactic treatment of nutritional and medical complications of HIV.

## Definitions of HIV and AIDS

The human immunodeficiency virus is a transmissible retrovirus that undergoes replication in human host cells and causes HIV infection, an asymptomatic immune infection that can lead to AIDS. Former names for HIV were human T-cell lymphotropic virus type III (HTLV-III), lymphadenopathy-associated virus (LAV), and AIDS-associated retrovirus. HIV is a retrovirus, so named because it must inject its RNA into its target cell and then transcribe the RNA into DNA (accomplished with a reverse transcriptase enzyme). Once DNA is created, it is then integrated into the host cell's DNA with the enzyme integrase. The host cell can become a factory for the replication of the virus. A protease enzyme then reconstructs the virus. From that point, the virus can "bud" from the host cell, destroying it in the process, and may infect other target cells and continue its life cycle. See Figure 1-1 for the life cycle of the virus and the effects of drug interventions at different stages.

The acquired immunodeficiency syndrome is a secondary immunodeficiency syndrome that results from infection by HIV. Currently, a diagnosis of AIDS does not mean that the disease is inevitably progressive. CD4 cell counts can even increase to normal levels. The acquired immunodeficiency syndrome is characterized by a diverse spectrum of disorders, including opportunistic infections, malignancies, neurologic dysfunctions, wasting, and gastrointestinal ailments.

The Centers for Disease Control and Prevention (CDC) define AIDS by the following (10):

- A positive antibody test for HIV.
- A CD4 cell count below 200/mm$^3$ or below 14% of the total white blood cell count (see the "Laboratory Indicators of HIV Infection" section in this chapter) *or*
- A clinical diagnosis of one of the 25 AIDS-defining diseases (Table 1-1).

#### TABLE 1-1  AIDS-Defining Diseases

**Bacterial Infections**
Salmonella septicemia, recurrent
*Mycobacterium avium* complex or *Mycobacterium kansasii,* disseminated or extrapulmonary
*Mycobacterium tuberculosis,* any site, pulmonary or extrapulmonary
*Mycobacterium* infections, other species or unidentified species, disseminated or extrapulmonary

**Cancers**
Kaposi's sarcoma
Lymphoma—Burkitt's (or equivalent term)
Lymphoma—immunoblastic (or equivalent term)
Lymphoma—primary, of brain
Cervical cancer, invasive

**Fungal Infections**
Candidiasis, pulmonary (trachea or lungs)
Candidiasis, esophageal
Coccidioidomycosis, disseminated or extrapulmonary (valley fever)
Cryptococcosis, extrapulmonary
Histoplasmosis, disseminated or extrapulmonary

**Protozoal Infections**
Isosporiasis, chronic intestinal (>1 month duration)
Cerebral toxoplasmosis
Cryptosporidiosis, chronic intestinal (>1 month duration)
*Pneumocystis carinii* pneumonia (PCP)

**Viral Infections**
Herpes simplex, chronic ulcers (>1 month duration); or bronchitis, pneumonitis, or esophagitis
Cytomegalovirus (CMV) retinitis (loss of vision)
CMV disease other than liver, spleen, or lymph nodes

**Other**
Neurological problems (encephalopathy)
Progressive multifocal leukoencephalopathy
Recurrent pneumonia
Wasting due to HIV

Source: Centers for Disease Control and Prevention. 1993 revised CDC HIV classification system and expanded AIDS surveillance definition for adolescents and adults. MMWR. Dec 18, 1992;41:RR-17.

**FIGURE 1-1  Life Cycle of HIV and Drug Intervention**

(1) HIV enters an uninfected cell. (2) Reverse transcriptase inhibitors can stop duplication of HIV's genetic material. (3) Without reverse transcriptase inhibitors, HIV's genetic material can get inside the cell's nucleus, its command center, where it makes long chains of proteins and enzymes into short chains. (4) Protease inhibitors can stop the cutting of long chains of HIV proteins and enzymes into short chains. (5) Protease inhibitors result in the formation of "empty" viruses that can't infect new cells. (6) Without protease inhibitors, short chains of HIV proteins and enzymes make new viruses that can infect other cells. Reprinted with permission from Markowitz M, *Protease Inhibitors: A New Family of Drugs for the Treatment of HIV Infection* (Chicago: International Association of Physicians in AIDS Care; 1996). Copyright © 1996 International Association of Physicians in AIDS Care.

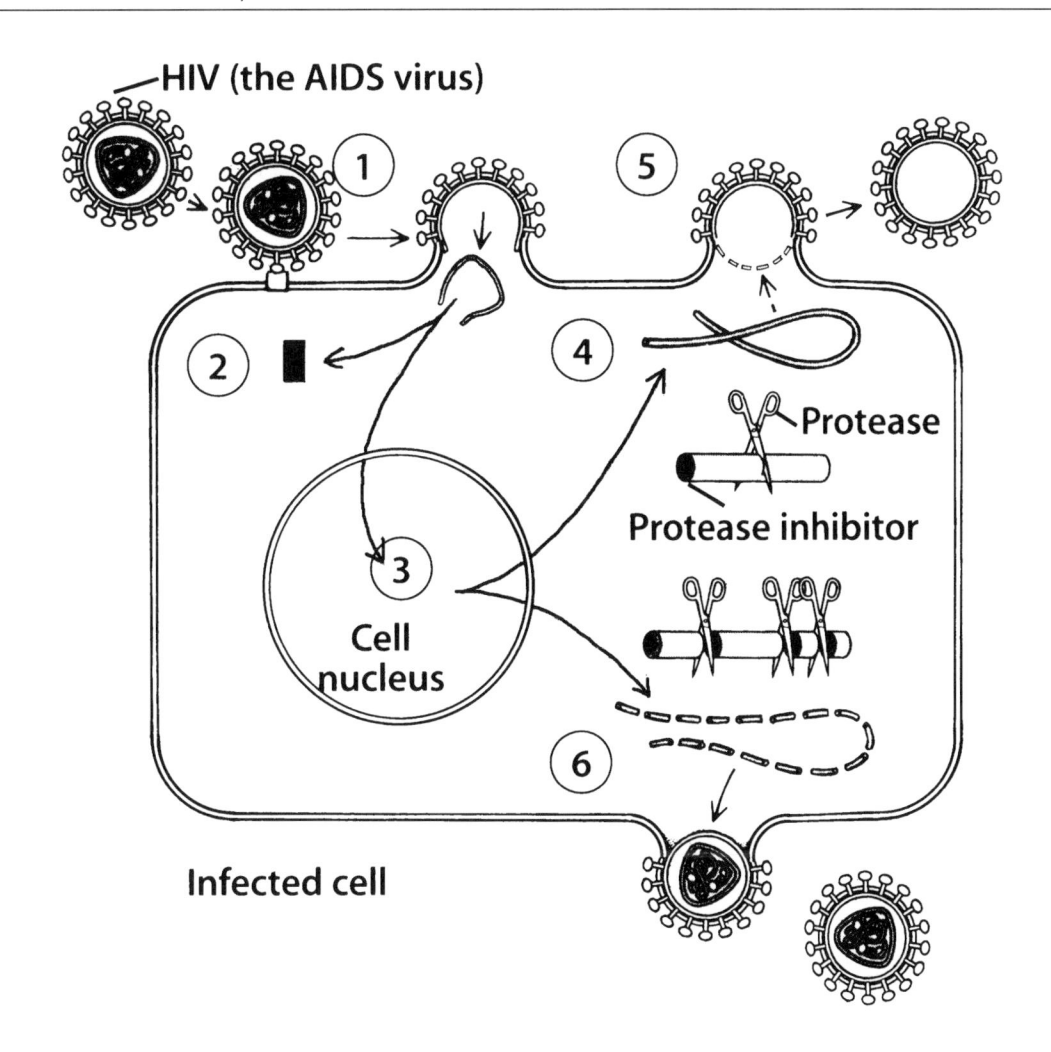

In developing countries where laboratory tests may not be available, the diagnosis of AIDS may rely solely on the clinical findings of the disease (11).

Previously, AIDS-related complex (ARC), a now outdated term, was used to explain the collection of chronic symptoms and signs indicative of HIV infection but without the opportunistic infections or tumors that define AIDS (12). One symptom of ARC and AIDS is wasting, or unintentional weight loss. In Africa, AIDS is termed "slim disease" because of the wasting that commonly occurs.

Being HIV positive does not necessarily mean that one has AIDS. HIV-positive status means that the results of the enzyme-linked immunosorbent assay (ELISA) and another laboratory test—Western Blot, polymerase chain reaction (PCR), or bDNA—confirm the presence of HIV antibodies or antigens (sometimes referred to as seropositive)(13).

As previously mentioned, two strains of HIV have been identified. The first strain, HIV-1, is more prevalent globally, whereas HIV-2 is found primarily in West Africa and also in East Africa, Europe, Asia, and Latin America (4). Both HIV-1 and HIV-2 have the same clinical manifestations and modes of transmission, although HIV-2 is much more virulent and life-threatening.

## Pathophysiological Process of HIV Infection

In humans HIV disables the immune system by infecting CD4 T cells that orchestrate immune function and macrophages that rid the system of infected cells, impairing immune response to everyday microorganisms. Eventually the virus disables target white blood cells of the immune system called T4 or CD4 lymphocytes. Other target cells singled out by HIV are B lymphocytes, monocytes, macrophages, and cells in other tissues in the body (13).

Often described in military terms, the virus stages a coup in the body and commandeers the T cells, ordering them to churn out genetic parts for the virus instead of the body (see Figure 1-1). After the manufacturing process is completed, new viral particles called virions (copies of the original HIV) are released from the T cell. The process of breaking out of the cell destroys it. A human infected with the virus can produce more than 1 billion copies of HIV every day. Several generations of HIV can be generated in a matter of hours.

The body continues to produce the virus throughout the course of HIV infection and appears to hold HIV level at an equilibrium, or set point. This equilibrium is different for each individual and may range from a few hundred to millions of copies of HIV. Although antiretroviral therapies may slow or halt destruction of the immune system, existing damage is poorly repaired. Restoration to a completely functioning immune system remains elusive.

Antibodies to HIV are usually detectable 2 to 4 months after exposure to HIV (13). Seroconversion means that the serum has changed from negative to positive, indicating that antibodies to HIV have been produced. At about this time, CD8 cells go into action and eliminate numerous infected cells. Throughout the asymptomatic stage of HIV infection, the levels of CD8 cells are high but can decrease if the disease progresses.

Under healthy conditions, the CD4 T cells are important players in the immune response that the body mounts to track down and kill invaders. But when the CD4 cell count decreases to a certain level, the body's immune system becomes vulnerable to fungi, parasites, bacteria, and viruses.

## Laboratory Indicators of HIV Infection

The CD4 cell count is a widely used marker of HIV disease progression (13). In healthy immune systems, the CD4 cell count typically ranges from 800 to 1,200/mm$^3$. When the count drops below 500/mm$^3$, the immune system is starting to weaken. When the CD4 count declines to 200/mm$^3$ and AIDS is officially diagnosed, some patients may become more open to opportunistic conditions such as infections and cancers.

The CD8 cells (suppressor T cells) destroy HIV-infected CD4 cells, so while the former is rising, the latter is falling. This ratio (CD4:CD8) is used to monitor the status of HIV infection (13). The CD8 cells' anti-HIV activity tends to weaken with time.

Another increasingly important immune marker is called viral load, which indicates the viral burden or amount of actual HIV in the body. This term is expressed as the number of RNA copies per milliliter (13). Health care providers are starting to use HIV viral load tests for evaluating HIV therapies, predicting the progression of HIV disease to AIDS, and assessing the efficacy of new antiviral medications (14). In an important study published in *Science* (15), researchers concluded that viral load predicts the risk for HIV disease progression to AIDS better than does the CD4 cell count. In 1996 another group of researchers released interim recommendations on the interpretation of viral load test results along with CD4 counts (Table 1-2). The higher the viral load, the greater the risk for clinical deterioration in HIV patients (14).

Roche Molecular Systems received approval from the FDA to market a viral load test called the reverse transcriptase PCR (RT-PCR) test, otherwise known simply as PCR. The Chiron Corporation also received approval from the FDA for another viral load test called the branched-chain DNA test, or bDNA. Both tests are expensive (up to $400 each), but competition and new testing strategies may reduce the price over time.

**TABLE 1-2  The Viral Load Test and CD4 Cell Counts: HIV Therapy Considerations**

| CD4 Count (per mm$^3$) | Viral Load (RNA copies per milliliter) | Treatment[a] |
|---|---|---|
| <350 | Any level | 2 nucleoside analogs[b] + protease inhibitor[c] |
| 350-500 | >5,000-10,000 | 2 nucleoside analogs + protease inhibitor to decrease viral load to <10,000 copies per milliliter |
| 350-500 | <5,000-10,000 | didanosine or stavudine[d] or 2 nucleoside analogs or observation |
| >500 | >5,000-10,000 | didanosine or stavudine or 2 nucleoside analogs or observation |
| >500 | <5,000-10,000 | observation or participation in clinical trials |

Source: Reprinted from *Beta*, a publication of the San Francisco AIDS Foundation. Used by permission.

[a]Another option is to treat all patients until viral load is below 10,000 copies per milliliter. Repeat the test 2-4 weeks later to obtain a baseline measurement.

[b]Nucleoside analogs include zidovudine (formerly AZT), didanosine (formerly dideoxyinosine, or ddI), zalcitabine (formerly dideoxycytidine, or ddC), stavudine (formerly d4T), and lamivudine (formerly 3TC). Two possible nucleoside analog combinations include (1) zidovudine + didanosine or zalcitabine or lamivudine or (2) stavudine + didanosine or lamivudine.

[c]Approved protease inhibitors include saquinavir, ritonavir, indinavir, and nelfinavir.

[d]Monotherapy with stavudine would be an option only after zidovudine has been tried.

## Modes of Transmission

Contaminated needles, tainted blood supplies, unprotected sex, and perinatal transmission are the major modes of HIV transmission. Transmission of the virus is possible only if the person has direct contact with bodily fluids containing infected cells. HIV may be transmitted in blood, semen, vaginal secretions, or breast milk.

Although HIV is present only in bodily fluids, the misinformation and fear surrounding the infection are as widespread as the disease itself. Some people may still fear airborne transmission of the virus or even a handshake from an HIV infected-person. Due to these erroneous fears, the late Ryan White could not attend public school in Indiana and Magic Johnson faced resistance to his playing professional basketball.

Certain risk behaviors increase the chance of contracting HIV. This is reflected in the kind of risk groups prevalent in the United States. High-risk categories, starting with the highest and decreasing in order, include recipients of blood transfusions; people using injectable drugs; those exchanging bodily fluids, as in anal and vaginal intercourse; and newborns of HIV-infected mothers. The prevalence of HIV may be proportionally higher in prisoners and prostitutes (13). For the most recent information on HIV transmission and risk categories, call the CDC's AIDS information hot line: 404/332-4565 and ask the Fax Information Service for Document No. 320210.

## Epidemiology

Worldwide, the AIDS epidemic has been estimated to affect 22.6 million people, 90% of whom live in developing countries (4). More than 6 million men, women, and children have died of AIDS (4,16). According to UNAIDS, a subgroup of the United Nations dedicated to AIDS (4), women account for 42% of the AIDS cases, and this number is climbing as the disease spreads among the heterosexual population in all countries. By the year 2000, the estimated number of infected women will be 15 million. In developing countries, HIV infection is increasing the fastest. Ninety percent of people with AIDS live in Africa, India, Latin America, and the Orient (4). In the United States, 1992 estimates of HIV prevalence ranged from 650,000 to 900,000 persons (17). Of these, 525,000 to 750,000 were men, and 120,000 to 160,000 were women; about 10,000 were children. Worldwide, approximately 1.5 million children have HIV infection, according to a World Health Organization estimate (4).

Although AIDS is rapidly growing in developing countries, its growth rate appears to be stabilizing in the United States and other developed countries (5). In the United States, AIDS is still increasing but more slowly than in years past (18). In 1995, 62,600 cases of AIDS were diagnosed in the United States, according to the CDC. This was only a 2% increase from the previous year, compared with a 5% increase between 1993 and 1994.

Despite the diminishing growth rate, the number of women with AIDS has increased. In 1995 AIDS was diagnosed in 9% (11,500) more women (primarily women of color) compared with 1994 (18). In contrast, the number of men diagnosed with AIDS increased less than 1% from 1994 to 1995.

## Clinical Manifestations of HIV Disease

At the onset of HIV infection, the person sometimes experiences rather severe flulike symptoms or a syndrome similar to mononucleosis for 2 to 4 weeks after exposure. This is usually followed by an asymptomatic period of 10 or more years. Some patients may rapidly progress to AIDS (19); this is especially true in developing countries where the asymptomatic period and survival time are shorter than in developed countries. However, as mentioned earlier, progression of the disease is not seen as inevitable. Viral load is sometimes used to predict disease progression. The theory is that if viral load is kept at an undetectable level, the disease should not progress.

Even during the asymptomatic stage, HIV is not dormant or latent in the body, as originally believed. HIV researchers Ho and colleagues (6) showed that the battle for control of the body may start at the beginning of the infection and continue relentlessly and systematically, even though this is not evident from the clinical profile of the patient, who appears to be healthy. This supports the "hit hard, hit early" philosophy of treatment, in which aggressive pharmacotherapy with nucleoside analogs and protease inhibitors aims at full suppression of viral replication. When HIV cannot replicate, viral resistance to any combination of drugs is prevented (20).

Symptoms of HIV disease progression may include fatigue, weight loss, body composition changes, and diarrhea. Other signs of disease progression are associated with opportunistic events. These may include night sweats, mouth sores, rashes, and fever.

Collectively, infections that are serious in immunocompromised, but not healthy, persons are known as opportunistic infections (Table 1-3). Two common opportunistic infections in people with AIDS in developed countries include PCP and *Mycobacterium tuberculosis* (11). These infections are rare in developing countries. Tuberculosis is a common AIDS-defining disease in Africa and increasingly is seen in the United States (11). Many opportunistic infections result from organisms in the patient's own body due to previous exposure.

Up to 60% of all persons with AIDS in developed countries have been affected by PCP (13). The drug therapies for PCP—pentamidine, a combination of trimethoprim and sulfamethoxazole (TMP/SMX), and dapsone—have helped prevent a higher incidence of this pneumonia.

Chronic diarrhea, fever, and wasting of body stores are characteristic symptoms of advanced HIV disease. Also, HIV can manifest itself neurologically, resulting in meningitis, peripheral neuropathies, encephalopathy with seizures, and dementia (12). At this stage of HIV disease, there may be an increased susceptibility to neoplasms such as Kaposi's sarcoma and non-Hodgkin's lymphoma.

No one dies of AIDS itself, but of diseases that develop as a result of a suppressed immune system. The most prevalent cause of death is a respiratory disorder, and the next most common is cancer (13). Mounting a strong immune response to HIV further depletes the body's

**TABLE 1-3  Opportunistic Infections**

| Complications | Site | Sample Symptoms | Sample Treatments[a] | Comments |
|---|---|---|---|---|
| Candidiasis | Mouth, vagina, esophagus, gastrointestinal (GI) tract, and/or skin | White coating on tongue | Fluconazole, ketoconazole, nystatin, oral clotrimazole troches | Commonly known as thrush; most common fungal infection in AIDS |
| Cervical cancer | Uterine cervix | Abnormal cervical cells on Pap smear | Excision, cryotherapy, electrosurgery, laser treatment, hysterectomy for invasive cancer | AIDS-defining condition for HIV-infected women |
| Cytomegalovirus (CMV) | Retina, colon, esophagus | Floaters (black spots floating in line of vision), altered vision | Retinal reattachment; foscarnet and ganciclovir | CMV is a herpesvirus; duration of therapy is lifelong |
| Coccidioidomycosis | Lungs | Cough, fatigue, weight loss | Fluconazole, amphotericin B, itroconazole | Fungus found in southwestern United States |
| Cryptococcal meningitis | Brain | Fatigue, fever, headache, nausea, seizures, neurologic dysfunctions | Amphotericin B and fluconazole | Yeastlike fungus in soil |
| Cryptosporidiosis | GI tract | Watery diarrhea, abdominal cramps, weight loss, anorexia, flatulence | No therapies have reliably palliated or cured. | Parasitic infection from fecal-infected water; individuals at risk are advised to boil tap water |
| Dementia | Central nervous system (CNS), peripheral nervous system | Decreased concentration and rapidity of thought, loss of interest, loss of short-term memory, slow motor movement | Treatment is based on cause; zidovudine (formerly AZT), pentoxifylline, peptide T, vit $B_{12}$, pyrimethamine | HIV has neurological implications in almost all infected persons; medications make a slight improvement |
| Diarrhea and malabsorption | Small intestine, large intestine, pancreas | Sporadic or continuing loose stools; fullness/bloating; abdominal pain | Reduced lactose, fat, and fiber; increased fluid and electrolyte intake; prescription pancrelipase therapy; antidiarrheal medications | Causes: GI abnormalities from HIV infection (short, atrophied villi), opportunistic infections, food-borne illnesses, drug-nutrient interactions, exocrine, pancreatic dysfunction |
| Hairy leukoplakia | Tongue, rectum, labia | White lesions that are corrugated and "hairy" | Topical podophyllin resin and/or high-dose acyclovir | Sign of advancing HIV disease |

## TABLE 1-3 Opportunistic Infections *(Continued)*

| Complications | Site | Sample Symptoms | Sample Treatments[a] | Comments |
|---|---|---|---|---|
| Herpes simplex virus (HSV)/ herpes zoster virus (HZV) | Nerve tissue, mouth and lips (HSV type 1), genitals and anus (HSV type 2), face and buttocks (HZV) | Painful oozing blisters | Acyclovir for treatment of HSV; acyclovir and famciclovir, foscarnet for HZV | HZV may manifest as shingles. |
| Histoplasmosis | Lungs, systemic | Fever; weight loss; skin lesions; respiratory problems; anemia; enlarged spleen, liver, and lymph nodes | Amphotericin B or itraconazole | Fungus in south-central United States and South America |
| Human papillomavirus (HPV) | Vagina, vulva, perianal area, anal canal, penis, urethra | Genital warts on the skin and mucous membranes | Electrocautery, cryotherapy, laser, radiation therapy | Caused by anogenital contact; more common in women; detected by a Pap smear |
| Coccidiosis (isosporiasis) | Intestines | Diarrhea, abdominal cramps, weight loss | Similar to cryptosporidiosis | Parasite in tropical and subtropical climates |
| Kaposi's sarcoma | Skin, GI tract, lungs | Red and purple lesions, edema | Cancer chemotherapy, radiation therapy, interferon alpha with ddI and interferon alpha with AZT, experimental GM-CSF and radiation, removal of lesions with liquid nitrogen | Most common malignancy in HIV infection |
| Lymphoma | Lymph nodes | Swollen lymph nodes | Chemotherapy or GM-CSF | Confirmed by biopsy; types are non-Hodgkin's lymphoma, CNS lymphoma, and Hodgkin's disease |
| *Mycobacterium avium* complex (MAC) | GI tract, almost any organ | Fever, night sweats, weight loss, weakness, anorexia, malabsorption, abdominal pain | Clarithomycin, azithramycin, TLC G-65, rifabutin, ciprofloxacin, amikacin | Bacteria found in food, soil, and water |

**TABLE 1-3  Opportunistic Infections  (Continued)**

| Complications | Site | Sample Symptoms | Sample Treatments[a] | Comments |
|---|---|---|---|---|
| Pelvic inflammatory disease (PID) | Uterus, fallopian tubes, ovaries | Vaginal discharge, pelvic pain, and pain during intercourse | Antibiotics | Usually transmitted by sexually transmitted microbes (e.g., gonococci and chlamydiae); PID can lead to infertility, ectopic pregnancy, and chronic abdominal pain; it is more common and severe in women with HIV |
| Peripheral neuropathy (polyneuropathy) | Peripheral nerves | Painful tingling and burning in the limbs, usually accompanied by edema | Peptide T, acupuncture with mexiletine (red chili pepper ointment) and amitriptyline (Elavil) | May occur as a medication side effect requiring dose or medication changes |
| *Pneumocystis carinii* pneumonia (PCP) | Lungs, spleen, lymph nodes, liver, bone marrow | Fever, dry cough, chest tightness, difficulty breathing | Trimethoprim and sulfamethoxazole (TMP/SMX) (Bactrim), pentamidine, or dapsone | Most common opportunistic infection; caused by a parasite |
| Progressive multifocal leukoencephalopathy (PML) | Brain | Speech and language deficits, nerve palsies, loss of vision, sensory loss on one side | No standard treatment | Rapidly progressive and fatal |
| Salmonellosis | GI tract | Diarrhea, fever, chills, weight loss, perspiration, anorexia | High-dose antibiotics: TMP/SMX, ciprofloxacin, ampicillin | Bacterial infection caused by eating or drinking contaminated water |
| Toxoplasmosis | Central nervous system | Headache, confusion, seizures, fever | Sulfadiazine, pyrimethamine, and clarithromycin for treatment; phenytoin (Dilantin) for seizure prevention | Protozoal disorder caused by ingesting raw or undercooked meat. |
| Tuberculosis (TB) | Lungs | Fever, weight loss, cough, night sweats, fatigue | Rifampin, isoniazid (INH), pyrazinamide, ethambutol | Bacterial infection that is common in HIV-infected persons with previous exposure to TB |
| Wasting syndrome | Full body | Involuntary weight loss >10% diarrhea >30 days, or fever >30 days | Dronabinol and megestrol acetate-testosterone, growth hormone, thalidomide, antiinflammatory drugs | — |

Source: Adapted from Abdale F. *Community-Based Nutrition Support for People Living With HIV and AIDS: A Technical Assistance Manual.* New York: God's Love We Deliver, 1995, appendix. Used by permission.
[a] ddI, dideoxyinosine (now called didanosine); GM-CSF, granulocyte-macrophage colony stimulating factor. Manufacturer information: Mycelex Troches, Bayer Pharmaceutical, West Haven, CT 06516; Elavil, Zeneca Pharmaceuticals, Wilmington, DE 19850; Bactrim, Roche Laboratories, Nutley, NJ 07110; Dilantin, Parke-Davis, Morris Plains, NJ 07950; and Megace, Bristol Myers Squibb Co, Princeton, NJ 08543.

protein. Skeletal muscle is used initially and then organ tissues are catabolized as a source of protein. This promulgates a vicious cycle of a weakened defense leading to infections, which in turn further depletes the protein resources of the body. With defenses compromised by malnutrition, pneumonia is commonly the immediate cause of death (21).

## Nutritional Implications of AIDS

An important job of the dietitian who works with patients with HIV and AIDS is to screen and assess their nutritional status (see Chapter 2). The major concerns of dietitians working with HIV-positive patients fall into two categories: nutrition as prevention of malnutrition and nutrition as therapy for malnutrition.

### CAUSES AND TYPES OF MALNUTRITION

Malnutrition has been observed during all stages of HIV infection (22). The causes of malnutrition include anorexia and inadequate intake, malabsorption and other gastrointestinal disorders, hypermetabolism, or alterations in metabolic response and food-drug interactions.

Although many types of malnutrition may occur, wasting syndrome is the most visible type. Wasting syndrome is defined by the CDC as a 10% unintentional loss in body weight, with either diarrhea for more than 30 days or weakness and fever for more than 30 days. The CDC added wasting syndrome to the list of AIDS-defining illnesses in 1987 (13) (see Table 1-1). Wasting in HIV disease begins with poor oral intake, which usually reflects an underlying problem such as a medical condition, depression, medication interaction, or lack of access to food (22).

### EFFECTS OF MALNUTRITION

A vicious cycle is operative in HIV infection. The infection can cause malnutrition, which contributes to additional immune dysfunction, leading to an opportunistic disease. This further jeopardizes the integrity of the immune response in the body (23).

Protein-energy malnutrition is a cofactor in the progression of HIV disease (20). In HIV, as in starvation or cancer, when the patient is at 66% of ideal body weight or 54% of total body potassium (an indicator of body cell mass), death is likely to occur (24).

Jain and Chandra (25) hypothesized that nutritional deficiencies are important in the pathogenesis of HIV. They observed many commonalties in immunologic parameters between AIDS and protein-energy malnutrition: T cells are decreased, the helper-suppressor T-cell ratio is inverted, lymphokine production and helper T-cell activity are decreased, many tests of cellular immune function are abnormal, and natural killer cell function is markedly decreased. Good nutritional status, according to Jain and Chandra, might provide the host with additional resistance to AIDS-related infections by preventing and/or reversing nutrition-related immune dysfunction.

Other effects of malnutrition in persons with HIV besides increased immune dysfunction and opportunistic diseases include diarrhea.

Diarrhea also may be caused by the HIV infection itself, drug-nutrient interactions, and gastrointestinal disease.

Even in healthy people, food-borne microorganisms can cause illness. The gastrointestinal tract begins with an oral cavity exposed to the elements and is therefore vulnerable to infections. Normally, the mucous membrane coating the gut serves as a barrier to viruses, parasites, bacteria, and fungi. When body proteins are depleted in the patient with HIV, the microvilli of the intestine may atrophy and become shortened and flattened (14). Foods cannot be absorbed, and malabsorption results. A disease of the gut (enteropathy) could also be caused by the viral infection itself. Diarrhea may further increase the damage. When the bowel becomes inflamed or the mucosa atrophies, malnutrition results.

## PREVENTION OF MALNUTRITION

Because food-borne and water-borne illnesses are particularly problems for patients with immunodeficiency and can lead to malnutrition, special care should be taken with food preparation and consumption. It is of utmost importance that patients with HIV learn about food safety to protect their fragile gastrointestinal tract and to prevent infections caused by unsafe food.

Guidelines to prevent food-borne and water-borne infections include the following:

- Keep cold foods cold and hot foods hot.
- Clean and sanitize the kitchen.
- Observe proper sanitary procedures when preparing, delivering, and serving food.
- Discard leftovers.
- Drink safe water or boil tap water.

Most public water systems do not test for *Cryptosporidium*, a protozoa that causes cryptosporidiosis, an illness with severe diarrhea, fever, and weight loss in immune-compromised patients. The CDC has issued advisories for patients to bring tap water to a rapid boil for 1 minute before drinking it. (See Chapter 3 for additional information.)

## TREATMENT OF MALNUTRITION

A field of study has focused on micronutrient alterations in HIV infection, notably vitamin A, beta carotene, vitamin E, ascorbic acid, riboflavin, folic acid, vitamin B-6, vitamin B-12, zinc, copper, and iron (23, 26, 27). Many of these alterations may be related to the body's stress response to infection or altered metabolism and may not be true deficiencies. Because more studies are needed to confirm whether intake of individual micronutrients would alter the course of HIV infection, many physicians and dietitians specializing in HIV disease are hesitant to recommend single micronutrients to their patients. Recommendations instead include healthy meals, a multivitamin and mineral supplement that meets from 100% to 200% of the US Recommended Daily Allowances (RDA) (or as individually prescribed), and possibly an oral supplement and appetite stimulant. Special diets, vitamin and mineral supplementation, and complementary therapies are all reviewed in Chapter 3.

After HIV infection is diagnosed, medical nutrition therapy should be included as an integral part of the ongoing health care of patients with HIV (28). The main thrust of nutrition therapy is to support and restore nutritional status. Gastrointestinal symptoms can be initially managed orally (see Chapter 3). Therapeutic diets are modified according to content (acid, fat, protein, fiber, salt, sugar, lactose), consistency (soft or pureed), portion size (kilocalories), and accompanying disease (diabetic or renal).

Early nutrition intervention for patients with AIDS has three objectives: to improve nutrition-related immune function, to support prevention of opportunistic infections, and to enhance response to therapy (26). Additionally, early nutrition intervention is important to preserve lean body mass (see Chapter 2) and improve the patient's mental attitude.

Diets need to be individualized because HIV disease is complex, with many different medical conditions to manage. If oral intake fails or is at risk of failing, then enteral and parenteral nutrition are the next options (see Chapter 4). Other pertinent responsibilities of the dietitian, ranging from the clinic to the community, are discussed in Chapter 5.

The psychological impact of malnutrition can be devastating. Malnutrition with wasting has a strong negative impact on self-esteem, precipitating isolation, depression, lack of appetite, and aversion to eating (29). Some persons are distressed with their physical deterioration and emaciated appearance. Recommended interventions may include individualized meal plans, food supplements, appetite stimulants, and anabolic strategies, such as exercise, medication, or both. By developing a meal plan in conjunction with the client, the dietitian supports the client's ability to exert control over his or her health. Eating can thus symbolize empowerment. When patients with HIV start to gain weight and look better, it can have a positive effect on their outlook, their ability to recover, and even their will to live (29).

## Summary

Although much has been learned about HIV and AIDS since the early 1980s, HIV infection is still an epidemic with serious consequences. Opportunistic infections, wasting syndrome, and cancer may occur frequently. Early nutrition intervention is important to preserve lean body mass, prevent infections, improve the patient's mental attitude, and enhance the response to therapies. Progress has been made in treating HIV infection, and infected individuals are living longer; however, management of HIV disease remains a challenge for the clinician.

## References

1. Lacayo R. Hope with an asterisk (CNN-*Time* Poll on Dec 11-12, 1996). *Time.* Dec 30-Jan 6, 1997, p 49.
2. Plague, *Microsoft Encarta Encyclopedia.* Redmond, Wash: Microsoft Corp, 1993-1995.
3. Wallbank TW, Taylor AM, Bailey NM, Jewsbury GF, Lewis CJ, Hackett NJ. *Civilization: Past & Present.* 6th ed. Glenview, Ill: Scott, Foresman; 1987:433-434.
4. UNAIDS and WHO. *The Global Epidemic,* December 1996. Based on *The Status and Trends of the Global HIV/AIDS Pandemic,* Vancouver, Canada, July 5-6, 1996 (http://www.who.gov).
5. Fauci AS. AIDS in 1996. Much accomplished. Much to do. *JAMA.* 1996;276:155-156. Editorial.
6. Ho DD, Neumann AU, Perelson AS, Chen W, Leonard JM, Markowitz M. Rapid turnover of plasma virions and CD4 lymphocytes in HIV-1 infection. *Nature.* 1995:373:123-126.
7. Barre-Sinoussi F, Chermann JC, Rey F, Nugeyre MT, Charmet S, Gruest J, Dauguet C, Axler-Blin C, Vezinet-Brun F, Rouzioux C, Rozenbaum W, Montagnier L. Isolation of a T-lymphotropic retrovirus from a patient at risk for acquired immune deficiency syndrome (AIDS). *Science.* 1983;220:868-871.
8. Blayney DW, Blattner WA, Jaffe ES, Gallo RC. Retroviruses in human leukemia. *Hematol Oncol.* 1983;1:193-204.
9. Bloom FE. Breakthroughs of the year, 1996. *Science.* 1996;274:1987. Editorial.
10. Osmond DH. Classification and staging of HIV disease. In: Cohen PT, Sande MM, Volberding PA, eds. *The AIDS Knowledge Base.* 2nd ed. New York, NY: Little, Brown; 1994:1-15.
11. Beach RS. Nutrition and HIV/AIDS in developing countries. In: *Nutrition and HIV/AIDS: Proceedings of the 1992 International Symposium on Nutrition and HIV/AIDS.* Vol. 1. Chicago, Ill: PAAC; 1992:43-51.
12. Berkow R, ed. *The Merck Index.* 16th ed. Rahway, NJ: Merck Research Laboratories;1992:77-96.
13. Casey KM, Cohen F, Hughes AM. *ANAC's Core Curriculum for HIV Nursing.* Philadelphia, Pa: Nursecom; 1996.
14. Baker R. HIV viral load testing. *San Francisco AIDS Foundation Newsletter.* July 1996.
15. Mellors JW, Rinaldo CR Jr, Gupta P, White RM, Todd JA, Kingsley LA. Prognosis in HIV-1 infection predicted by the quantity of virus in plasma. *Science.* 1996;272:1167.
16. Mertons TE, Burton A. Estimates and trends of the HIV/AIDS epidemic. *AIDS.* 1996;10(suppl A):S221-228.
17. Karon JM, Rosenberg PS, McQuillan G, Khare M, Gwinn M, Peterson LR. Prevalence of HIV infection in the United States, 1984 to 1992. *JAMA.* 1996;276:126-131.
18. Henderson C. AIDS slowing but not among women and blacks. *AIDS Weekly Plus.* Nov 11, 1996, p 10.
19. Timbo BB, Tollefson L. Nutrition: a cofactor in HIV disease. *J Am Diet Assoc.* 1994;94:1018-1022.
20. Deeks SG. New principles of HIV-related medical care. *Focus: A Guide to AIDS Research and Counseling.* 1997;12:5-7.
21. Stein TP. Effect of HIV on metabolism and the relationship to muscle and body protein content. In: Watson RR, ed. *Nutrition and AIDS.* Ann Arbor, Mich: CRC Press; 1994:167-188.
22. Nutrition management of HIV infection and AIDS. In: The Chicago Dietetic Association and The South Suburban Dietetic Association: *Manual of Clinical Dietetics.* 5th ed. Chicago, Ill: The American Dietetic Association; 1996:381-394.
23. Bradley-Springer L. Nutritional support in HIV infection: a multilevel analysis. *IMAGE: J Nurs Scholarship.* 1991;23:153-159.
24. Nerad JL, Gorbach SL. Nutritional aspects of HIV infection. In: Management of Infection in HIV Disease. *Infect Dis Clin North Am.* 1994;8:499-515.
25. Jain VK, Chandra RK. Does nutritional deficiency predispose to acquired

immune deficiency syndrome? *Nutr Res.* 1984;4:537-643.
26. Abrams B, Duncan D, Hertz-Picciotto IH. A prospective study of dietary intake and acquired immune deficiency syndrome in HIV-seropositive homosexual men. *J AIDS.* 1993;6:949-958.
27. Beach RS, Mantero-Atienza E, Shor-Posner G, Javier JJ, Szapocznik J, Morgan R, Sauberlich HE, Cornwell PE, Eisdorfer C, Baum MK. Specific nutrient abnormalities in asymptomatic HIV-1 infection. *AIDS.* 1992;6:701-708.
28. Position of The American Dietetic Association and The Canadian Dietetic Association: nutrition intervention in the care of persons with human immunodeficiency virus infection. *J Am Diet Assoc.* 1994;94:1042-1045.
29. Weaver KE. Psychosocial aspects pertaining to nutrition. In: Kotler DP, ed. *Gastrointestinal and Nutritional Manifestations of AIDS.* New York, NY: Raven Press;1991:279-294.

# 2
# Nutrition Screening and Assessment

The position article on the human immunodeficiency virus (HIV) and the acquired immunodeficiency syndrome (AIDS) issued by The American Dietetic Association and The Canadian Dietetic Association states that medical nutrition therapy "should be an integral part of the ongoing health care of people with HIV" (1). This therapy should begin shortly after HIV is diagnosed. First, the patient should receive a screening for general risk factors indicating a poor nutritional status and then should undergo a thorough nutrition assessment conducted by or under the supervision of an HIV-knowledgeable dietitian.

Monitoring the outcome of nutritional care is another priority of the dietitian. Because medical nutrition therapy for HIV and AIDS is a relatively new specialty that is evolving, knowledge gaps exist in finding the most appropriate assessment tools. This chapter is intended as a starting point for exploring what is available today to help clinicians do a better job of screening and assessing the nutritional status of patients with HIV and AIDS.

## Nutrition Screening

### DEFINITION

Medical nutrition therapy involves the assessment of the nutritional status of patients with a condition, illness, or injury that puts them at risk for nutritional deficiencies. Nutrition therapy includes review and analysis of the patient's medical and diet history, laboratory values, and anthropometric measurements (1). Nutrition screening, the first step, can be defined as a process to pinpoint dietary or nutritional problems. The purpose is to identify persons at high risk of nutritional problems or who already present with poor nutritional status (2). Once the individuals at high risk have been identified, a thorough nutrition assessment is needed to indicate the type of therapy necessary to resolve or ameliorate the problems.

Many of the risk factors and indicators of malnutrition in HIV disease may be identified by well-designed nutrition screenings in most clinical and community settings. Tools developed for nutrition screening in HIV disease share the same characteristics as tools used in other disease states (2).

Level I screening, based on the comprehensive model set forth in the Nutrition Screening Initiative (3), may be conducted by a patient or other layperson (Figure 2-1). If "alerts" occur at this stage, such as the patient lost 10 lb or more in the last 6 months, a level II screening (Figure 2-2) is necessary to provide more specific data on nutritional status. A level II screening needs to be conducted by a dietitian or other qualified health professional.

## REFERRAL DATA

Before a dietitian schedules an initial session with an HIV-infected patient, as much referral information as possible should be obtained. The patient's confidentiality must be ensured, and a consent to release medical nutrition information between a dietitian and primary care physician or facility is required.

The first step in determining the current nutritional status of the patient includes obtaining the following information (4):

1. Results of laboratory tests for albumin, prealbumin, blood (serum) urea nitrogen (BUN), creatinine, electrolyte, cholesterol, and triglyceride levels; complete blood cell count (CBC); and CD4 and CD8 cell counts and viral load, if available.

---

**FIGURE 2-1  Level I Nutrition Screening Adapted for HIV Disease**

**Body Weight**
Height (in):_____  Weight (lb)_____
❏ Weight change: has lost 10 lb or more in the last 6 months

**Dietary Problems**
❏ Poor appetite
❏ Has difficulty chewing
❏ Has difficulty swallowing
❏ Has pain in mouth, teeth, or gums
❏ Has gastrointestinal problems
❏ Unable to secure or prepare food
❏ Has more than one alcoholic drink a day
  (if a woman); more than two drinks a day (if a man)

**Living Environment**
❏ Lives on an income of less than $6,000 per year
  (per individual in the household)
❏ Lives alone
❏ Is homebound
❏ Does not have a stove or refrigerator

**Functional Status**
Usually or always needs assistance with:
❏ Eating
❏ Preparing food
❏ Shopping for food or other necessities

*Place a check by any statements that are true for the individual. If you have checked one or more statements on this screening, the individual you have interviewed may be at nutritional risk; please complete level II screening assessment.*

Source: Based on the level I nutrition screening from the Nutrition Screening Initiative. Reprinted with permission of the Nutrition Screening Initiative, a project of the American Academy of Family Physicians, The American Dietetic Association, and the National Council on the Aging, Inc, and funded in part by a grant from the Ross Products Division, Abbott Laboratories.

## FIGURE 2-2 Level II Nutrition Screening Adapted for HIV Disease

**Anthropometrics**
Height (in) _____    Weight (lb) _____    Body mass index (BMI): _____
Weight change[a]: has lost 10 lb or more or 5% of body weight in the past 6 months _____
Midarm circumference (MAC) (cm): _____ (record to nearest 0.1 cm)
Triceps skinfold (TSF) (mm): _____ (record to nearest 2 mm)
Check any abnormal values:
❑ Midarm muscle circumference (MAMC) below 10th percentile[a]
❑ TSF below 10th percentile[a]

**Laboratory Data[b]**
❑ Serum albumin level below 35 g/L[a]
❑ Serum cholesterol level below 4.14 mmol/L
❑ Triglyceride level above 2.82 mmol/L
CD4 cell count (mm$^3$) _____    Viral load ____ detectable ____ undetectable

**Drug Use**
❑ Three or more prescription drugs, over-the-counter (OTC) medications, or vitamin and mineral supplements daily[c]
List prescribed drugs _____
List OTC medications _____
List vitamin and mineral supplements _____
List alternative therapies _____

**Clinical Features[c]**
❑ Anorexia                   ❑ Esophagitis (inflamed esophagus)    ❑ Stomatitis (inflamed mouth)
❑ Diarrhea                   ❑ Gingivitis (swollen gums)           ❑ Candidiasis (thrush)
❑ Dysgeusia (altered taste)  ❑ Nausea and vomiting                 ❑ Xerostomia (dry mouth)
❑ Dysphagia                  ❑ Odynophagia (painful swallowing)
  (difficulty swallowing)

**Eating Habits[c]**
❑ Does not have enough food to eat each day          ❑ Has one or no serving of milk or milk products daily
❑ Usually eats alone                                  ❑ Has one or no serving of fruit or fruit juices daily
❑ Has poor appetite                                   ❑ Has five or fewer servings of bread and grain products daily
❑ Is on a special diet (specify) _____      ❑ Has more than one alcoholic drink a day (if a woman);
  _____                more than two alcoholic drinks a day (if a man)
❑ Eats two or fewer servings of vegetables daily

**Activities of Daily Living (ADL)**
❑ Unable to secure or prepare food[a]          Usually or always needs assistance with[a]:
❑ Lives alone                                   ❑ Eating                    ❑ Grooming
❑ Has no stove or refrigerator                  ❑ Food preparation/shopping ❑ Toilet
❑ Unable or prefers not to spend money on food  ❑ Bathing                   ❑ Walking or moving about

Source: Based on the Level II Nutrition Screen from the Nutrition Screening Initiative. Reprinted with permission of the Nutrition Screening Initiative, a project of the American Academy of Family Physicians, The American Dietetic Association, and the National Council on the Aging, Inc, and funded in part by a grant from the Ross Products Division, Abbott Laboratories.

[a] Major risk factor or indicator of poor nutritional status. Patients in whom you have identified one or more major indicators need immediate medical attention.

[b] To convert g/L albumin to g/dL, multiply g/L by 0.1. To convert mmol/L cholesterol to mg/dL, multiply mmol/L by 38.7. To convert mmol/L triglycerides to mg/dL, multiply mmol/L by 88.6.

[c] Minor risk factor or indicator of poor nutritional status. Patients with minor indicators or other risk factors should be referred to appropriate health care professionals, such as a physician, nurse, social worker, dietitian, or case manager.

2. Clinical signs and symptoms such as fever or sweats, dehydration, early satiety, diarrhea, voluntary energy expenditure, skin disorders, muscle pain, non-life threatening opportunistic infections, and abnormal bowel habits.
3. The referring physician's goals for nutrition intervention and overall health care plan.
4. The patient's medical history and family medical history.
5. Medication regimen (including prescription and over-the-counter drugs and self-prescribed vitamin, mineral, and herbal supplements).
6. Alternative or complementary therapies that the patient uses (see Chapter 3).
7. Performance status, activities of daily living (see Figure 2-2), and living situation.

For more information, see Appendix B for the revised HIV/AIDS Medical Nutrition Therapy (MNT) Protocol.

## Stages of HIV Infection

Infection with HIV may not be a progressive disease for persons who are able to control and manage it. Although HIV infection is believed to be permanent, a decrease in and vigilant monitoring of viral load may help an infected person remain asymptomatic for up to his or her lifetime.

The Centers for Disease Control and Prevention (CDC) define HIV infection in three clinical categories (see Table 2-1 for definitions). Additional scales used to stage HIV infection or define function include the Walter Reed Staging Classification for HIV Infection and the Karnofsky Scale (see Appendix B).

The first condition in primary HIV infection is acute retroviral syndrome (ARS), which causes flulike symptoms when seroconversion occurs. Not all persons infected with HIV experience ARS. After ARS, HIV is identified in clinical categories according to the CDC. Clinical category A is an asymptomatic stage, but nutrition intervention is important at the onset. Nutrition intervention will ensure an adequate diet, correct any misinformation that the patient may have, and, through baseline measurements, address hidden symptoms, such as a decreased lean body mass (LBM) with no accompanying decrease in weight or a vitamin B-12 deficiency (5). The three important roles of early nutrition intervention in HIV infection are: to prevent or forestall lean tissue wasting; to improve the efficacy of medical therapies; and to positively influence clinical, functional, and psychological well-being (5).

Currently, if a patient progresses toward more symptomatic categories, proper medical and adjunctive care can actually cause a regression toward an asymptomatic status. Antiretroviral therapy is aimed at keeping viral load in check because higher levels of virus are associated with symptoms, reduced CD4 cell counts, disease progression, and mortality. Each person appears to react differently to how the body reacts to and reproduces HIV. After primary infection with HIV, the body settles into an equilibrium or "set point" when the virus replicates enough to keep a certain level or titer in the blood (6, 7).

## CLINICAL CATEGORY A

In the first category, an HIV-positive person is seemingly asymptomatic or may have persistent generalized lymphadenopathy. Clinical evidence of immune deficiency has not surfaced, and an important laboratory marker of immune dysfunction, the CD4 cell count, may be at any level (see Table 2-1). A CD4 cell count of less than $200/mm^3$ in clinical category A is defined as AIDS (A3; see Table 2-1).

## CLINICAL CATEGORY B

The patient becomes symptomatic in category B, and again the CD4 cell count can vary (Table 2-1). Again, AIDS (B3) is defined as a CD4 cell count less than $200/mm^3$(8).

## CLINICAL CATEGORY C

The diagnosis of AIDS is made when any of the 26 AIDS-defining conditions are present (see Table 1-1). All patients in category C qualify for the diagnosis of AIDS. The CD4 cell count may or may not be below $200/mm^3$ as in categories A and B.

# Medical Nutrition Therapy Protocols

The initial nutrition session is the time to collect baseline data on anthropometric measurements, biochemical values, nutrition and medical history, nutrient intake (adequacy of the diet), and clinical findings (4). Other factors to assess during this stage are lifestyle and psychosocial issues, exercise patterns, use of vitamins and minerals, alternative nutrition treatments, medication use, alcohol consumption, and smoking habits.

One or two follow-up sessions a year are also needed to take measurements, such as weight, triceps skinfold (TSF), midarm muscle circumference (MAMC), and bioelectrical impedance analysis (BIA); identify new dietary problems; and provide strategies to support medications and other therapies, which will help keep the patient symptom free. At this time, preventive education can be provided about basic nutrition, health maintenance, and food and water safety (see Chapter 3).

The dietitian needs to monitor those parameters addressed in category A, note any change in weight and LBM, review the patient's food record, determine if any HIV symptoms are contributing to nutrition-related problems such as diarrhea or dysphagia, and encourage an appropriate diet (see Chapter 3). The initial session should last 30 to 60 minutes, with two to six shorter follow-up visits scheduled as needed each year (4).

Nutritional care essentially covers the same variables as in the other two categories; however, the level of complications often increases. Nutrition assessment involves taking anthropometric measurements and a nutrition history as well as recording clinical symptoms. Food intake is evaluated for levels of calories, protein, fat, fluids, lactose, and fiber. Dietary supplementation, exercise and activity, substance use, and

### TABLE 2-1 Classifications of HIV Disease

The revised system emphasizes the importance of CD4 lymphocyte testing in clinical management of HIV-infected persons. The system is based on 3 ranges of CD4 cell counts and 3 clinical categories, giving a matrix of 9 exclusive categories. The system replaces the 1986 classification.

| CD4 Cell Level | Clinical Category | | |
|---|---|---|---|
| (1) >500/mm$^3$ | A1 | B1 | **C1** |
| (2) 200-500/mm$^3$ | A2 | B2 | **C2** |
| (3) <200/mm$^3$ | **A3** | **B3** | **C3** |

Bold letters indicate categories reportable as AIDS effective January 1, 1993. Categories A3 and B3 were previously not reported as AIDS.

**Clinical Category A**
Asymptomatic HIV infection
Persistent generalized lymphadenopathy (PGL)
Acute (primary) HIV illness

**Clinical Category B**
Must be attributed to HIV infection or have a clinical course or management complicated by HIV
Symptomatic (not A or C conditions) including but not limited to:
  Bacillary angiomatosis
  Candidiasis, vulvovaginal: persistent longer than 1 month, poorly responsive to prescribed therapy
  Candidiasis, oropharyngeal
  Cervical dysplasia, severe, or carcinoma in situ
  Constitutional symptoms (eg, temperature above 38.5˚C or diarrhea longer than 1 month)

**Clinical Category C**
Presence of an AIDS-defining condition including:
  Candidiasis: esophageal, trachea, bronchi
  Coccidioidomycosis, extrapulmonary
  Cervical cancer, invasive
  Cryptosporidiosis, chronic intestinal (duration >1 month)
  Cytomegalovirus retinitis
  HIV encephalopathy
  Herpes simplex with mucocutaneous ulcer present longer than 1 month, bronchitis, pneumonia
  Histoplasmosis: disseminated, extrapulmonary
  Isosporiasis, chronic (duration >1 month)
  Kaposi's sarcoma
  Lymphoma: Burkitt's, immunoblastic, primary, of brain
  *Mycobacterium avium* or *Mycobacterium kansasii,* extrapulmonary
  *Mycobacterium tuberculosis,* pulmonary or extrapulmonary
  *Mycobacterium,* other species disseminated or extrapulmonary
  *Pneumocystis carinii* pneumonia
  Pneumonia, recurrent (>2 episodes in 1 year)
  Progressive multifocal leukoencephalopathy
  Salmonella bacteremia, recurrent
  Toxoplasmosis, cerebral
  Wasting syndrome due to HIV

Source: Centers for Disease Control and Prevention. 1993 revised CDC HIV classification system and expanded AIDS surveillance definition for adolescents and adults. *MMWR.* Dec 18, 1992;41:RR-17.

smoking patterns are also reviewed. The dietitian needs to devote the same amount of time for counseling in this category as in category B. The patient may be at increased risk for complications. During acute events the patient may require more intensive monitoring. Aggressive interventions such as enteral or parenteral nutrition (see Chapter 4) are sometimes required. For more on the protocols, see Chapter 5.

## Nutrition Assessment

Nutrition assessment can be defined as a procedure for gathering data about current nutritional status and adequacy of the diet. The data must be interpreted to identify any problems contributing to malnutrition, determine the degree of malnutrition if present, and develop an individualized nutrition care plan (5).

Protein-energy malnutrition and other types of malnutrition have a detrimental effect on immune function. Immune dysfunction can contribute to disease and further compromise nutritional status. There is much evidence to show that cachexia, protein-energy malnutrition, and severe weight loss are prevalent in HIV-infected patients (9-11). Hence, the goals of nutrition assessment and intervention are to improve the nutritional status, enhance the quality of life, and prolong survival (12).

Important components of an in-depth nutrition assessment include the following: anthropometric measurements, biochemical values, drug-nutrient interactions, and clinical findings. Assessment also should include a review of the patient's medical history and psychosocial background.

### ANTHROPOMETRIC MEASUREMENTS

*Height, Weight, and Body Mass Index*

Height should be measured by clinical personnel because self-reports may be inaccurate. An accurate measurement of height is essential to appropriate evaluation and individualized nutrition care planning. Height should be noted as a "measured height" to differentiate it from and to correct self-reported height where necessary. Standardized methods for measuring height and weight are shown in Appendix B.

Measured weight can vary widely from scale to scale and according to the patient's attire. Accurate serial measurements should be made on the same scale. The patient's weight needs to be measured and recorded at every visit.

One of the criteria for diagnosing AIDS used by the CDC is involuntary weight loss greater than 10% from baseline, with concomitant diarrhea or fever over a period of 1 month (13). In one study on the relationship between weight maintenance and the course of HIV infection (14), the researchers found that weight loss was independently prognostic of clinical outcome; the more weight lost, the sicker the patients became. Weight losses have been estimated to occur in up to 80% to 90% of patients during the course of HIV disease (15). The dietitian, in counseling the HIV-infected patient about weight loss, must evaluate the dietary adequacy, eating patterns and habits, and swallowing difficulties and odynophagia; assess concurrent gastrointestinal problems and opportunistic infections such as candidiasis, cytomegalovirus, and herpes simplex virus; and provide strategies to gain or maintain weight, if needed.

Reasons for weight loss vary. They include decreased caloric intake due to anorexia or oral and esophageal lesions, malabsorption due to intestinal damage or pancreatic dysfuntion, and altered metabolism due to chronic infection. One problem in using weight loss as an indicator of malnutrition in HIV and AIDS is that body cell mass (BCM), a component of LBM most associated with survival, may be decreased with no change in weight (16).

A quick method for estimating ideal body weight (IBW) is as follows (5):

- Males: 106 lb for the first 5 ft of height plus 6 lb per inch over 5 ft or minus 6 lb per inch under 5 ft.
- Females: 100 lb for the first 5 ft of height plus 5 lb per inch over 5 ft or minus 5 lb per inch under 5 ft.
- Large-framed persons: Add 10% to the above calculations.
- Small-framed persons: Subtract 10% from the above calculations.

When evaluating an HIV-infected patient's nutritional status, it may be more appropriate to use the patient's reported usual body weight (UBW), although it is still important to monitor IBW. Usual body weight is defined as the weight that one attains by age 21 and maintains for most of one's adult life.

The percentage of IBW, UBW, and weight loss over time (Figure 2-3) are important data for the dietitian to collect in all staging categories of HIV and AIDS (4). Because unintentional weight loss is sometimes the first symptom of HIV infection (15), dietitians specializing in HIV and AIDS care must recognize these warning signs of malnutrition. Typically, a weight 85% to 95% of UBW indicates mild depletion, 75% to 84% of UBW reflects moderate depletion, and below 75% represents severe depletion. Significant weight loss is 5% of UBW in 1 month and 10% in 6 months (5). Research into HIV disease suggests that weight loss of 5% or greater is associated with increased morbidity and mortality (17).

Height and weight measures are used to establish a body mass index (BMI), defined as weight in kilograms over height in meters

---

**FIGURE 2-3  Calculation of Percentages of Ideal Body Weight (IBW), Usual Body Weight (UBW), and Weight Change**

$$\% \text{ IBW} = \frac{\text{Current Body Weight}}{\text{IBW}} \times 100$$

$$\% \text{ UBW} = \frac{\text{Current Body Weight}}{\text{UBW}} \times 100$$

$$\% \text{ Weight Change} = \frac{\text{UBW} - \text{Current Body Weight}}{\text{UBW}} \times 100$$

squared. Using the chart in Appendix B, the clinician can determine BMI, which indicates body weight and also assesses health risk and the relationship of body fat and weight to morbidity and mortality (5). A BMI of 20 to 25 is normal. Health risks increase as BMI falls under 20, although BMI does not identify changes in LBM or BCM (18).

*Skinfold Measurements*

Skinfold measurements, which estimate the level of subcutaneous fat, total body fat, and somatic protein stores, include the following: midarm circumference (MAC), TSF, and MAMC.

**Midarm Circumference** The MAC is measured in centimeters on the upper arm. It determines skeletal muscle mass (somatic protein stores) and body fat stores (5). See Appendix B for measurement procedures.

**Triceps Skinfold** The TSF measurement estimates subcutaneous fat at one site and correlates closely with total body fat or degree of caloric deprivation. The thickness of a skinfold over the triceps muscle midway between the shoulder and the elbow on the back of the arm is measured (19). Then the values are compared with percentile values for age, gender, and race (see Appendix B). If the TSF is at or below the fifth percentile, the patient is considered to be malnourished (18, 19). One way to evaluate nutritional status is to collect TSF measurements over time during regularly scheduled check-ups. These could be monthly or annually, depending on disease status and goals for nutritional rehabilitation (5). Total body fat is estimated using multiple skinfold measurements.

**Midarm Muscle Circumference** Derived from the MAC and TSF values, MAMC (Figure 2-4) approximates muscle mass. Still one other indicator of protein-energy malnutrition is the upper arm muscle area (UAMA) (see Figure 2-4). Repeated measurements of somatic protein allow the clinician to determine changes in muscle mass over time (19).

*Biochemical Impedance Analysis (BIA)*

Body cell mass, mainly muscle protein, is the key factor to monitor in health maintenance. When BCM losses are at 46%, death is inevitable (6). Depletion of BCM is greater in patients with chronic diarrhea compared with those without diarrhea (15). Assessment of total body protein is dif-

---

**FIGURE 2-4 Calculation of Midarm Muscle Circumference (MAMC) and Upper Arm Muscle Area (UAMA)**[a]

$$\text{MAMC (cm)} = \text{MAC (cm)} - [3.14 \times \text{TSF (cm)}]$$

$$\text{UAMA (mm}^2\text{)} = \frac{[\text{MAC (mm)} - (\text{TSF (mm)} \times 3.14)]^2}{4 \times 3.14 \text{ (or 12.57)}}$$

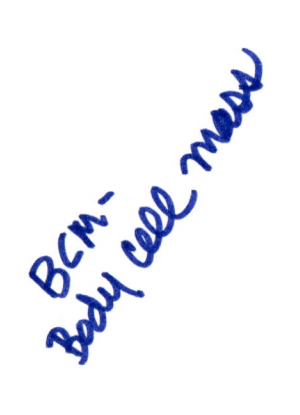

[a] MAC indicates midarm circumference; TSF, triceps skinfold. MAMC value derived from the formula is multiplied by 10 to convert to millimeters and is compared with standards.

ficult because the measurements are invasive, inconvenient to the subject, and somewhat costly. Only neutron activation analysis, which is not done in a clinical setting, measures protein stores directly (20).

An estimate of body composition can be achieved in the clinical setting by BIA. There are several types of BIA hardware on the market, along with many versions of software to evaluate body compartments. The primary endpoint of interest that BIA can monitor is lean tissue, specifically BCM. A three-compartment model of body composition allows for monitoring shifts in fluids and muscle. In this model, the body is divided into three parts: BCM, extracellular mass (ECM) or extracellular tissue (ECT), and fat mass. Body cell mass is primarily made up of highly functional protein stores (eg, muscles and organs). When BCM increases or decreases, the changes are attributed to mostly muscle tissue. Extracellular mass is made up of less calorie-intensive tissues such as bone, collagen, and plasma. When ECM increases or decreases, it may be primarily fluid shifts, including edema or fluid response to infection. Bioelectrical impedance analysis can help assess whether weight changes are due to shifts in BCM or ECM, thereby helping the clinician to more carefully monitor rehabilitation goals. Since BCM is more closely correlated with survival than the more general category of LBM, the three-compartment model more sensitively estimates the success of medical therapies (21-23). See Figure 2-5 for BIA evaluation measures using the optimal weight of BCM and the BCM-to-ECT ratio.

In addition to the above measures, phase angle values are also used to evaluate BIA measurements. Phase angle is a reflection of the ratios of body compartments. A phase angle can be reduced if BCM drops or ECM and fat increase. Increased phase angle calculations may reflect either an increase in BCM or a reduction in ECM or fat. A phase angle of less than 4.8 has been associated with an increased risk of morbidity and mortality(24). Though the phase angle provides an interesting overview, evaluation of calculated BCM is more essential to medical decision making.

Additionally, BIA is useful in measuring short-term fluid changes due to infections or changes in hydration status, and in conditions in which a major disturbance of body water occurs. A two-compartment model of body composition differentiates lean from fat tissues without

---

**FIGURE 2-5 Bioelectrical Impedance Evaluation of Body Cell Mass (BCM) and BCM-to-Extracellular Tissue (ECT) Ratio**

**BCM**
Males: Optimal Weight of BCM = Ideal Body Weight x 0.42
Females: Optimal Weight of BCM = Ideal Body Weight x 0.32

Calculation: Actual Weight of BCM ÷ Optimal Weight of BCM
= Percentage of Optimal BCM

**BCM-ECT Ratio**
Calculation: BCM ÷ ECT

Males: Optimal BCM:ECT Ratio~1.0
Females: Optimal BCM:ECT Ratio~0.9

separating out BCM and ECM. Results for both two- and three-compartment models for BIA have been compared with more sophisticated measures of body composition analysis, with comparable results (25).

Guidelines for conducting single-frequency BIA measurements and a sample BIA report are in Appendix B. Although the following factors do not significantly affect a clinical evaluation, clinical research BIA protocols may require the subjects to do the following before the test to ensure precise measurements(26):

- Avoid vigorous exercise 24 hours before the test.
- Fast for at least 8 hours before the test.
- Do not drink alcoholic beverages 24 hours before the test.
- Drink at least 1.5 liters of liquid 24 hours before the test.
- Urinate within 30 minutes before each measurement.

Although both single-frequency and multifrequency BIA machines are available, the former have demonstrated adequate accuracy in a clinical setting, are more compact, and produce more consistent results. The multifrequency machines may be more costly and have not evolved for ease of use in clinical settings at this time.

## BIOCHEMICAL VALUES

### Laboratory Values

Lack of nutrients, use of medications, and illnesses associated with metabolic alterations—all affecting patients with HIV infection—may alter biochemical values, so results need to be interpreted cautiously (5). Another problem is that virtually no laboratory values have been firmly established as normal or expected in HIV disease.

Because of the potential of protein tissue wasting in patients, visceral protein measurements represent the most helpful laboratory indicators of nutritional status. Serum albumin is the most widely used indicator of nutritional status (5); its levels reflect chronic protein depletion (19). Patients with normal serum albumin tend to live longer than those whose albumin levels are low (12, 27). Nevertheless, dehydration can increase plasma albumin, leading to false-negative values (20), whereas infection and edema can decrease plasma albumin, regardless of nutritional status (5). Malabsorption and the use of steroids can also affect levels of this visceral protein. Still, sample criteria for identifying protein-energy malnutrition can be useful documentation and includes albumin levels and a weight-to-height ratio (28) (Table 2-2).

Other important indicators of protein status include prealbumin and transferrin (see Table 2-2). Prealbumin is more sensitive than albumin or transferrin for reflecting the short-term effectiveness of medical nutrition therapy (5, 27). Prealbumin is sensitive as an indicator of visceral protein status, particularly in acute protein-energy malnutrition (19). In one study (29), transferrin and retinol-binding protein were better markers of malnutrition than albumin. Functioning as a carrier protein for iron, transferrin is a "more sensitive indicator of nutritional status than albumin and more reflective of acute changes" (19). Retinol-binding protein is clinically significant because it also shows acute

### TABLE 2-2  Malnutrition Assessment

| Laboratory Value[a] | Normal | Mild | Moderate | Severe |
|---|---|---|---|---|
| Prealbumin (mg/L) | 200-500 | 100-150 | 50-100 | <50 |
| Albumin (g/L) | 35-50 | 28-34 | 21-27 | <21 |
| Transferrin (g/L) | >2 | 1.5-2 | 1-1.5 | <1 |
| Creatinine-height index (%) (actual/ideal x 100) | 80-100 | 60-80 | 40-60 | <40 |
| Ideal body weight (%) | 90-100 | 80-90 | 70-80 | <70 |
| Usual body weight (%) | 95-100 | 85-95 | 75-85 | <75 |

Sources: Hickey MS. *Handbook of Enteral, Parenteral, and ARC/AIDS Nutritional Therapy.* Chicago, Ill: Mosby Year Book; 1992; *Manual of Clinical Dietetics.* 5th ed. Chicago, Ill: American Dietetic Association; 1996.

[a]To convert mg/L prealbumin to mg/dL, multiply mg/L by 0.1. To convert mg/L retinol-binding protein to g/L, multiply mg/L by 0.001. To convert g/L albumin to g/dL, multiply g/L by 0.1. To convert g/L tranferrin to mg/dL, multiply g/L by 100.

changes in protein malnutrition (kwashiorkor). Each of these laboratory values is affected by an acute phase response and by the metabolic dysfunction that sometimes occurs in HIV disease. (See Table 2-3 for ICD-9 diagnostic codes for malnutrition.)

Other laboratory values suggested for assessment (4) include creatinine-height index (a measurement of somatic protein), cholesterol, triglycerides, BUN, electrolytes, liver enzymes, zinc, selenium, vitamins A and B-12, iron, testosterone (total and free), and CBC. A CBC provides information on the total number of white and red blood cells present. In addition, a differential cell count breaks out types and levels of white blood cells. Triglyceride values are increased as a normal immune scavenger function, but cholesterol levels are decreased because liver metabolism may be altered (14). Very low cholesterol levels have been associated with increased morbidity and mortality in HIV disease, as in other

### TABLE 2-3  Nutrition-Related ICD-9 Codes

| ICD-9 Code | Diagnosis | Definition |
|---|---|---|
| 260 | Kwashiorkor | Protein deficiency with dyspigmentation of skin and hair |
| 261 | Nutritional marasmus | Nutritional atrophy, severe calorie deficiency, severe malnutrition not otherwise specified (NOS) |
| 262 | Other severe protein-energy malnutrition | Nutritional edema without mention of dyspigmentation of skin and hair |
| 263.0 | Malnutrition of moderate degree | — |
| 263.1 | Malnutrition of mild degree | — |
| 263.9 | Unspecified protein-energy malnutrition | Dystrophy due to malnutrition and protein-energy malnutrition NOS |
| 799.4 | Cachexia | Wasting disease, excluding nutritional marasmus |

Source: *St. Anthony's Softbound ICD-9-CM Code Book for Physician Payment.* Vols 1 and 2. Reston, Va: St. Anthony Publishing; 1996.

diseases (18). Medications, such as some antiretroviral agents, may cause an increase in both triglyceride and cholesterol levels in some persons. In these cases, dietary intervention may be ineffective.

## Drug-Nutrient Interactions

Drug therapies may change the interpretation of laboratory values. For instance, use of the antiretroviral zidovudine (formerly AZT) may result in a macrocytosis that does not necessarily indicate folate or vitamin B-12 deficiency. Rifampin, an antitubercular medication, can interfere with folate and vitamin B-12 status. Therefore, appropriate interpretations of deficiencies require a search for additional factors. Anemia is another problem resulting from the use of several drugs, including zidovudine, foscarnet, dapsone, and pyrimethamine.

Each medication should be evaluated for potential nutritional consequences (Table 2-4). Some medications indirectly affect nutritional status. An example is the appetite stimulant megesterol acetate (Megace, Bristol Myers Squibb Co, Princeton, NJ 08543). While improving appetite and yielding weight gain (mostly fat), megesterol may compromise testosterone balance in some men, making it difficult to maintain and efficiently restore BCM.

Some common side effects of medications commonly taken by HIV-infected patients are dry mouth, diarrhea, nausea, vomiting, and anorexia (see Table 2-4). Also, some of these medicines may make food taste strange. Strategies for coping with these problems are presented in Chapter 3.

Combination drug therapy, whereby one drug acts in combination with another drug to produce a synergistic effect, is determined to be more effective in treating HIV infection than is monotherapy. For example, the action of the antiviral medication zidovudine is enhanced if used together with didanosine (formerly dideoxyinosine, or ddI), lamivudine (formerly 3TC), or zalcitabine (formerly dideoxycytidine, or ddC)(30). Three kinds of drugs are currently being used to treat asymptomatic HIV disease: antiretroviral drugs (non-nucleoside reverse transcriptase inhibitors, nucleoside reverse transcriptase inhibitors, and protease inhibitors), immune modulators (eg, interferon, which increases the CD4 cell count), and prophylactic drugs against opportunistic infections. Recent developments in HIV therapeutics and monitoring have changed the attitude in the medical community from pessimism to optimism with the advent of more effective drug combinations and viral load testing.

Combination therapies reduce viral load and decrease the incidence of morbidity and mortality (31). Special care must be taken to reduce unwanted food-drug interactions that lead to drug resistance and failure of therapy. A dietitian can assist in meal planning, timing of medications, and food composition, to help increase tolerance to drugs while reducing unwanted side effects.

Foods and nutrients can affect the absorption and metabolism of HIV drugs. For example, the bioavailability of saquinavir, a protease inhibitor, increases after a high-energy, high-fat meal (54 to 57 g of fat) (32). It may be helpful to add a high-fat nutritional supplement to a meal

TABLE 2-4  Potential Drug-Nutrient Interactions of Medications Commonly Used in HIV Disease

| Category of Use | Medication[a] | Potential Side Effects | Potential Drug-Nutrient Interactions/Recommedations |
|---|---|---|---|
| Reverse transcriptase inhibitors | zidovudine (AZT) (Retrovir) | Anemia, nausea, hypertriglyceridemia, hepatomegaly, anorexia, vomiting, weight gain, altered taste, dyspepsia, elevated liver function tests (LFT), diarrhea, fever | High-fat meal may decrease peak plasma concentrations; take with low-fat meal |
| | didanosine (dideoxyinosine, or ddI) (Videx) | Hyperglycemia, diabetes mellitus, hypertriglyceridemia, diarrhea, abdominal pain, nausea, anemia, hepatomegaly, bloating, peripheral neuropathy (10%), pancreatitis (5%): more common with history of heavy alcohol intake or hepatitis, elevated LFT, increased serum amylase (often of salivary origin) | Take at least 1/2 hour before or 2 hours after meals |
| | zalcitabine (dideoxycytidine, or ddC) (HIVID) | Oral ulcers, dysphagia, abdominal pain, constipation, hepatomegaly, anemia, peripheral neuropathy (up to 25%), pancreatitis (<3%), nausea, diarrhea, anorexia, vomiting, myalgia, fatigue, weight loss | Absorption decreases with food; take without food |
| | stavudine (d4T) (Zerit) | Nausea, vomiting, abdominal pain, diarrhea, pancreatitis (<3%), increased serum glutamate pyruvate transaminase (SGPT), peripheral neuropathy (15%-21%), elevated LFT | Absorption decreases 45% with food but systemic availability is unaffected; take without regard to food |
| | lamivudine (3TC) (Epivir) | Nausea (33%), fatigue (27%), diarrhea (18%), vomiting (13%), anemia, neuropathy (12%), anorexia (10%), fever and chills (10%), abdominal pain (9%), dyspepsia (5%), extreme caution advised in administering to pediatric patients with a history or risk of pancreatitis (14%), elevated LFT | Take without regard to food |
| | abacavir succinate (BW 1592U89) | Nausea, headache, asthenia, rash | — |
| | nevirapine (Viramune) | Nausea, fever, elevated LFT; weight loss (2%) | No diet restrictions |
| | delaverdine (Rescriptor) | Abdominal pain and distention, anorexia, aphthous ulcers, colitis, constipation, diarrhea, intestinal inflammation, dry mouth, pancreatitis, anemia | Take without regard to food |
| Protease inhibitors | indinavir sulfate (Crixivan) | Nausea, vomiting, abdominal pain, diarrhea, fatigue, nephrolithiasis (5%), asymptomatic elevated bilirubin (10%), pharyngitis, taste changes | Adequate hydration is crucial to prevent kidney stones; drink >1.5 liters of fluid; take 1 hour before or 2 hours after meals; may take with nonfat light snack |

**TABLE 2-4  Potential Drug-Nutrient Interactions of Medications Commonly Used in HIV Disease (Continued)**

| Category of Use | Medication[a] | Potential Side Effects | Potential Drug-Nutrient Interactions/Recommedations |
|---|---|---|---|
|  | ritonavir (Norvir) | Nausea; vomiting; diarrhea; abdominal pain; anorexia; taste changes; dyspepsia; hyperlipidemia; gastrointestinal (GI) distress; abdominal pain; elevated LFT, triglycerides, cholesterol GGT, creatine phosphokinase (CPK), and uric acid | Take with meals; may need to mask taste |
|  | saquinavir mesylate (Invirase) | Diarrhea, abdominal discomfort, nausea, hypoglycemia, increased CPK, mild GI complaints, caution advised in patients with hepatic insufficiency, photosensitivity, elevated LFT | Recommended 54-57 g of fat in meal with dose; meal effect persists up to 2 hours; take within 2 hours of high-fat meal; taken without food, drug levels are too low |
|  | nelfinavir mesylate (Viracept) | Mild to moderate diarrhea, nausea, flatulence, abdominal pain | Take with meal or light snack |
| Antifungal | amphotericin B (Fungizone) | Nausea, vomiting, anorexia, metallic taste, abdominal pain, decrease in glomerular filtration rate (GFR), nephrocalcinosis, hypokalemia, hypomagnesemia, anemia, weight loss, sore throat | — |
|  | flucytosine (Ancobon) | Nausea, vomiting, diarrhea, anorexia, anemia, hepatotoxicity | — |
|  | ketozconazole (Nizoral) | Nausea, vomiting, abdominal pain, diarrhea, hepatotoxicity, decreased testosterone and corticosteroid synthesis, reversible adrenal insufficiency, abnormal liver function test results | Gastric acid required for absorption |
| Antibacterial | isoniazid (Nydrazid) | Increased need for pyridoxine, folate, niacin, and magnesium; hepatitis; constipation; anemia; fatigue | Flushing after ingesting Swiss cheese; may decrease absorption of pyridoxine, calcium, and vitamin D |
|  | rifampin (Rifadin, Rimactane) | GI irritation, anemia, jaundice, pancreatitis, altered taste, anorexia | May interfere with folate and vitamin B-12 levels |
|  | clarithromycin (Biaxen) | Diarrhea, abnormal taste, abdominal pain | Take without regard to food |
| Antiprotozoal | dapsone (Dapsone USP) | Nausea, vomiting, oral lesions, hemolytic anemia if glucose-6- phospate dehydrogenase (G6PD) deficient, anorexia, abdominal pain | Take on empty stomach if possible |
|  | paromomycin sulfate (Humatin) | Nausea, abdominal cramps, diarrhea | — |
|  | pentamidine isethionate (Pentam 300) | Nausea, vomiting, nephrotoxicity, pancreatitis, hypocalcemia, hypoglycemia followed by hyperglycemia | — |

TABLE 2-4  Potential Drug-Nutrient Interactions of Medications Commonly Used in HIV Disease (Continued)

| Category of Use | Medication[a] | Potential Side Effects | Potential Drug-Nutrient Interactions/Recommedations |
|---|---|---|---|
| | trimethoprim and sulfamethoxazole (Cotrim, Bactrim, Septra) | Bone marrow suppression, hyperkalemia, diarrhea, stomatitis, hepatitis, increased serum creatinine and BUN, abnormal liver function test results | Decreased absorption of folate and vitamin K; increased urinary excretion of vitamin C |
| Antiviral | acyclovir (Zovirax) | Occasional diarrhea, fatigue, sore throat, increased serum creatinine, abnormal liver function test results, hematuria, nausea, altered taste | — |
| | ganciclovir (Cytovene) | Anemia, renal impairment, fever | Take with high-fat meal |
| Immune modulator | interferon alpha (Intron A, Alferon N) | Anorexia, diarrhea, fatigue | — |

Sources: Sanford JP, Sande MA, Gilbert DN, Gerberding JL. *The Sanford Guide to HIV/AIDS Therapy*. Dallas, Tex: Antimicrobial Therapy Inc;1994; Fields Newman C, Horn B. *Drug-Nutrient Interactions in AIDS Guidebook*. Cary, Ill: The Cutting Edge; 1988; Moore Allen A. *Powers and Moore's Food Medication Interactions*. 8th ed. Pottstown, Pa: Food-Medication Interactions;1993; Bahl S. Drug-induced nutritional complications and their management. In: Bahl S, Hickson JF Jr: *Nutritional Care for HIV-Positive Persons: A Manual for Individuals and Their Caregivers*. Ann Arbor, Mich: CRC Press; 1995.

[a]Manufacturer information: Abacavir, Retrovir, Septra, Epivir, and Zovirax, Glaxo Wellcome, Research Triangle Park, NC 27709; Videx, Fungizone, Zerit, and Nidrazid, Bristol Myers Squibb Co, Princeton, NJ 08543; HIVID, Invirase, Bactrim, Ancobon, and Cytovene, Roche Laboratories, Nutley, NJ 07110;Viramune, Roxane Laboratories, Columbus, OH 43228; Rescriptor, Pharmacia & Upjohn, Kalamazoo, MI 49001; Crixivan, Merck & Co, West Point, PA 19486; Norvir, Abbott Laboratories, Abbott Park, IL 60064; Viracept, Agouron Pharmaceuticals, La Jolla, CA 92037; Nizoral, Janssen Pharmaceutica, Titusville, NJ 08560; Isoniazid tablets, DuraMed Pharmaceuticals, Cincinnati, OH 45213; Rifadin, Hoechst Marion Roussel, Kansas City, MO 64134; Rimactane, Ciba-Geigy Corp, Summit, NJ 07901; Biaxin, Abbott Laboratories, Abbott Park, IL 60064; Dapsone USP, Jacobus Pharmaceutical Co, Princeton, NJ 08540; Humatin, Parke-Davis, Morris Plains, NJ 07590; Pentam 300, Fujisawa USA, Deerfield, IL 60015; Cotrim, Teva Pharmaceuticals USA, Sellersville, PA 18960; Intron A, Schering-Plough Corp, Kenilworth, NJ 07033; and Alferon N, Purdue Frederick Co, Norwalk, CT 06850.

(eg, ScandiShake, Scandipharm Inc, Birmingham, AL 35242, which has 30 g of fat with whole milk, or NuBasics Plus Drink, Nestle (Deerfield, IL 60015), which has 15.6 g of fat) (32). Conversely, HIV drugs such as isoniazid, nystatin, and octreotide can alter absorption of nutrients.

Another protease inhibitor, indinavir, needs to be taken on an empty stomach for absorption and with plenty of fluids to prevent kidney stones. The best time to take this drug is 1 hour before a meal or 2 hours after eating. Some side effects of indinavir include taste alterations, nausea, and vomiting. When a patient must receive indinavir in combination with didanosine, meal planning and adherence become more difficult because both drugs must be ingested on an empty stomach but cannot be taken together. Because didanosine is buffered, it would decrease absorption of indinavir. Indinavir must be taken every 8 hours to maintain drug levels in the blood. A recommendation may be to eat a nutritious meal, wait 2 hours, take the indinavir, wait 1 hour, take the didanosine, wait another hour, and then eat another good meal (28). It becomes obvious that education on timing of medications and meals and snacks is crucial for drug efficacy and maintenance of nutritional status.

## CLINICAL FINDINGS

An assessment of all the clinical signs and symptoms with nutritional implications in HIV-infected patients is a challenge because of the sheer number and variety of gastrointestinal problems inherent in this disease (Table 2-5). Gastrointestinal complaints may be common in persons with opportunistic infections. A survey suggested that up to 85% of patients with AIDS had GI complaints (33). For nutrition management of these problems, see Chapter 3.

Many HIV-infected patients experience malabsorption of nutrients, which, along with poor dietary intake and metabolic problems, leads to malnutrition (5). For this reason vitamin B-12 injections are often recommended. Total fat can also be reduced to less than 50 g or a medium-chain triglyceride (MCT) supplement provided if at all possible (4). Physician-ordered pancreatic enzymes and bile-sequestering powders are two other forms of treatment.

**TABLE 2-5  Common Gastrointestinal Problems in HIV Disease**

| Problem | Comments |
| --- | --- |
| Anorexia | Loss of appetite due to opportunistic infections or medications (eg, acyclovir for herpes simplex virus, pyrazinamide for *Mycobacterium avium* complex) |
| Oral candidiasis (thrush) | Types: angular cheilitis (red ulcers around the corner of the mouth), atrophic candidiasis (red lesions on the roof of the mouth and back of the tongue), and pseudomembranous candidasis (thrush: white patches on the oral mucosa of the mouth) |
| Dysgeusia | Altered sense of taste caused by certain drugs, severe zinc deficiency, and protein-energy malnutrition |
| Xerostomia | Dryness of the mouth caused by an enlarged salivary gland, certain medications, and opportunistic infections |
| Odynophagia | Painful swallowing of food caused by oral ulcers and oral and esophageal candidiasis |
| Dysphagia | Difficulty in swallowing; found in non-Hodgkin's lymphoma, and Burkett's lymphoma |
| Malabsorption | Symptoms include bloating, fullness, diarrhea, and steatorrhea |
| Diarrhea | Caused by certain medicines and food-borne bacteria (eg, *Salmonella, Shigella,* and *Campylobacter* species; *Mycobacterium avium-intracellulare*), non-Hodgkin's lymphoma and Burkett's lymphoma, cytomegalovirus, HIV, and protozoa (eg, *Cryptosporidum* species, *Isospora belli,* microsporidia, *Giardia lamblia*) |
| Nausea and vomiting | Due to drug-nutrient interactions, non-Hodgkin's lymphoma, Burkett's lymphoma, and food-borne illnesses |
| Gingivitis | Inflammation of the gums, sometimes seen in Kaposi's sarcoma |
| Stomatitis | Sore mouth and painful ulcers |
| Esophagitis | Inflammation of the esophagus caused by esophageal reflux, certain medications, and opportunistic infections |

In advanced disease many symptoms arise from opportunistic infections caused by microorganisms that take advantage of a severely compromised immune system. Diseases develop that normally do not affect a person with an intact immune system. One example of an opportunistic infection, which is the leading cause of death in HIV-infected patients, is *Pneumocystis carinii* pneumonia (PCP). Aerosolized and intravenous (IV) pentamidine has been used for treatment of PCP, but this medication is expensive and inconvenient (34). For this reason, many physicians specializing in HIV recommend trimethoprim and sulfamethoxazole (Bactrim, Roche Laboratories, Nutley, NJ 07110, or Septra, Glaxo Wellcome, Research Triangle Park, NC 27709) and dapsone; these medications stop the microbes from growing but may induce side effects such as nausea, vomiting, fever, rash, and anemia (34). Desensitization techniques allow patients to take this therapy even if they experience an allergic response.

It is often difficult to diagnose opportunistic infections because the cause is frequently multifactorial. Also, symptoms of the same disease vary from one patient to the next. The variety of medications and their reactions also complicates diagnosis and treatment. However, prompt and effective treatment is the first line of defense to prevent weight loss and a reduction in BCM (1, 35).

Fever and night sweats frequently affect patients who are infected with *Mycobacterium avium* complex (MAC) (34). Because these symptoms (and many medications) can cause dehydration, adequate fluid intake is especially important. Caffeinated or alcoholic beverages should be avoided and do not count toward fluid requirements because they can further increase fluid losses. Severe diarrhea is a hallmark of parasites such as *Cryptosporidium,* which causes the AIDS-defining infection cryptosporidiosis. This parasite may be present in tap water. Immune-compromised patients should drink distilled water, use filters, or boil water for 1 minute at a rapid boil to kill the microorganisms (18). Education on safe food, water, and sanitation practices by HIV-infected persons and their caregivers, as well as the public, is vital to reduce the incidence of diarrhea and dehydration, hospitalization, and mortality.

Evaluation of clinical signs of nutrient deficiency is an important part of overall nutrition assessment, although many signs are nonspecific. Physical examination may include observations of skin, hair, nails, eyes, and the oral cavity and an overall view of body dimensions (Table 2-6). From a formal examination to informal observations, a nutrition screening can identify potential problems that should be explored further through analysis of nutrient intake, laboratory evaluation, and review of nutrient-drug interactions and disease signs and symptoms.

## NUTRIENT INTAKE

Usual methods of nutrient intake analysis are presented in Table 2-7 according to their advantages and disadvantages. Three-day food diaries and weighed food records may be used in research settings with motivated patients. It is likely that 24-hour recalls or 24-hour usual intake records, along with a cross-check of food frequency records done

### TABLE 2-6  Physical Signs of Malnutrition

| Body Area | Physical Signs | Possible Deficits |
|---|---|---|
| Tongue | Filiform papillary atrophy | Iron, folic acid, riboflavin, niacin, B-complex vitamins |
|  | Fissuring, edema | Niacin |
|  | Lobulated with atrophy | Folic acid |
|  | Scarlet, raw, painful | Niacin, folic acid; possibly riboflavin or other vitamin B complex |
|  | Surface: bald, smooth, and beefy red | Niacin |
| Gums | Bleeding or red, swollen; interdental gingival hypertrophy | Ascorbic acid |
|  | Inflammation, stomatitis, ulceration | Ascorbic acid, folic acid, riboflavin |
| Lips/mucous membranes | Inflammation, angular scars, cheilosis, vertical fissuring, ulceration | Riboflavin |
|  | Pallor | Iron |
| Skin | Decubitus ulcers, delayed healing | Ascorbic acid, zinc, protein; possibly linoleic acid |
|  | Dry, rough, scaling; possibly with headache, diplopia, and dizziness | Excess vitamin A |
|  | Follicular hyperkeratosis | Vitamin A, ascorbic acid, linoleic acid |
|  | Hyperpigmentation | Protein energy, folic acid, riboflavin |
|  | Perifollicular petechiae (small hemorrhages around follicles) | Ascorbic acid; possibly vitamin A, linoleic acid |
|  | Petechiae other than perifollicular | Vitamin K |
|  | Pitting edema | Protein energy |
|  | Reduced turgor, tenting | Water, fluids |
|  | Seborrheic inflammation with erythema, thickening, dry, flaky | Linoleic acid, riboflavin |
|  | Subcutaneous ecchymosis (bruise) with minor trauma | Vitamin K, ascorbic acid, protein energy |
| Eyes | Corneal vascularization | Riboflavin, other vitamin B-complex factors |
|  | Dull, dry conjunctiva, Bitot's spots | Vitamin A |
|  | Pallor of everted lower eyelids | Iron, folic acid |

### TABLE 2-6  Physical Signs of Malnutrition (Continued)

| Body Area | Physical Signs | Possible Deficits |
|---|---|---|
| Hair | Broken, coiled, swan neck hairs, perifollicular hemorrhages, follicular hyperkeratosis | Ascorbic acid, vitamin A |
|  | Easily, painlessly pluckable; dry; brittle; lusterless | Protein energy, zinc |
| Nails | Pale, spoon shaped (koilonychia), ridging, brittle, thin, lusterless | Iron |
|  | Splinter hemorrhages under nails in semicircle lattice in nail bed | Ascorbic acid |
|  | White spotting | Zinc |

by an experienced interviewer, will give a reasonable overview of meal patterns as well as intake of macronutrients and micronutrients. In an institutional setting, records of calorie counts may be helpful to establish intake of macronutrients and even micronutrients.

Nutrient intake analysis of these records may be completed quickly using food group lists such as the Food Guide Pyramid or diabetic exchanges (Figure 2-6) or computerized programs designed to analyze nutrients. These records can be compared with estimated nutrient needs and the evaluation can be used in conjunction with other assessment factors to determine risk levels for malnutrition and appropriate goals for nutrition support.

## Review of Medical and Social History

A review of the medical history by interviewing the patient and reviewing his or her medical chart should reveal the following information: diagnoses, review of systems, presence of a chronic illness, medications, use of recreational drugs, tobacco, caffeine, alcohol, bowel habits, and surgical history (5).

The psychosocial aspects of patients with HIV and AIDS, which can evoke prejudice in some people, are considerable. The patient may have had a change in familial and social relationships and job, so the economic status must be ascertained. The dietitian should also know about family support, living situation, cooking facilities, and food assistance, if applicable (4). The patient's educational background and degree of literacy can affect how the dietitian provides information to that person. Ethnic and religious beliefs have an influence on food choices. Constructing dietary regimens compatible with the patient's dietary beliefs that are beneficial or neutral is important to successful nutrition intervention (36).

## Importance of Exercise

An exercise program that includes resistance training should be used by people with HIV to enhance and maintain muscle mass. Since a desir-

## TABLE 2-7 Methods of Dietary Intake Evaluation

| Method | Procedures | Comments |
| --- | --- | --- |
| 24-hour recall | Interview of previous day intake; may use food models and prompts to assist recall; identifies 24-hour intake of previous day only | Pros: fast and inexpensive<br>Cons: requires memory and ability to accurately report; requires experienced interviewer; may not represent usual intake |
| Food frequency | Interview or survey of food intake over a period (day, week, month); identifies food patterns | Pros: fast, inexpensive, and low burden<br>Cons: less accurate than food diaries; qualitative and not quantitative data |
| Diet history | Interview of 24-hour recall and usual intake; may include food frequency | Pros: cross-checks for data<br>Cons: requires memory and ability to accurately report; requires experienced interviewer; labor intensive |
| Estimated or weighed food records | Patient or caretaker records of actual intake over a period of 1 or more days; estimates are made by patient or caregiver | Pros: more accurate than other methods (depends on the recorder's skill and motivation)<br>Cons: expensive and time consuming; requires literate and motivated persons; high burden for patient or caretaker |

Source: Adapted from Gibson RS. *Principles of Nutritional Assessment*. New York, NY: Oxford University Press;1990:52. Used with permission.

able behavioral outcome of the HIV/AIDS MNT Protocol is to participate in resistance exercise to maintain LBM, dietitians should encourage the practice of weight lifting and other forms of resistance exercise with their clients (4).

Progressive resistance training (PRE) is a technique in rehabilitation medicine for increasing muscle strength (37). Repetitions, frequency, and intensity of training all have an influence on muscular strength. The effect of PRE on muscle function was studied in 24 male patients with AIDS (38). The experimental group did PRE three times a week for 6 weeks, and the control group did not exercise. The control group lost muscle mass and body weight in contrast to the PRE group, which gained weight and increased muscle mass.

Hand-grip dynamometry provides a baseline assessment of skeletal muscle function, although it may be influenced by patient motivation (19) (see Appendix B for a description of the procedure). Measurements are expressed as a percent of standard: $34.4 \pm 4.7$ kg for women and $48.8 \pm 7.0$ kg for men. An increased risk of morbidity and mortality is associated with less than 85% of the standard (22, 39).

It is not clear whether aerobic exercise suppresses or enhances the immune system (20). However, aerobic exercise is an important part of a rounded exercise program to improve endurance and muscle function. If patients infected with HIV are not accustomed to strenuous exercise, they should ease into an exercise program. They need to talk with an HIV-knowledgeable physician, physical therapist, or exercise physiologist about the type of exercise that is appropriate for their condition.

## FIGURE 2-6  Personal Nutrition Worksheet

My height: 5 feet = 60 in; 6 feet = 72 in  _____ in

My current weight:  _____ lb

Fluids I need each day: 1 c for every 15 lb of current weight:

_____ lb (current weight) ÷ 15 = _____ cups

Calories I need each day: males: 16 Calories per pound; females: 13 Calories per pound

Males: _____ lb (current) x 16 = _____ Calories

Females: _____ lb x 13 = _____ Calories

Protein I need each day for building muscle tissue (this is included in the food groups):

_____ Calories x 0.0416 = _____ grams of protein

### Servings per Calorie Level

| Food Group | 1,200 | 1,400 | 1,600 | 1,800 | 2,000 | 2,200 | 2,400 | 2,600 | 2,800 | 3,000 | 3,200 | 3,400 | 3,600 |
|---|---|---|---|---|---|---|---|---|---|---|---|---|---|
| Grains | 4 | 5 | 6 | 8 | 9 | 10 | 11 | 12 | 14 | 15 | 16 | 18 | 19 |
| Fruit | 4 | 4 | 4 | 4 | 4 | 4 | 4 | 4 | 4 | 4 | 4 | 4 | 4 |
| Vegetables | 3 | 3 | 3 | 3 | 3 | 3 | 3 | 3 | 3 | 3 | 3 | 3 | 3 |
| Dairy | 2 | 2 | 2 | 2 | 2 | 2 | 2 | 3 | 3 | 3 | 3 | 3 | 3 |
| Protein foods | 2 | 2.5 | 3 | 3 | 3 | 3.5 | 3.5 | 4 | 4.5 | 5 | 6 | 6 | 6 |
| Other | | | | | | | | | | | | | |

| Food Group | Serving Size | Comments |
|---|---|---|
| Grains | 1 slice bread, 1/2 bagel or English muffin<br>1 small tortilla, 1/2 hamburger bun<br>1/2 c cooked rice, pasta, cereal, or potatoes<br>4-6 crackers | Good source of carbohydrates, calories, and B vitamins; whole grains are a source of iron, magnesium, selenium, and zinc |
| Fruit | 1/2 c cooked or canned fruits<br>1/2 c fruit juice<br>1 c raw fruit | Good source of vitamins and minerals, especially antioxidants; follow food safety guidelines in washing raw fruit |
| Vegetables | 1/2 c of cooked vegetables<br>1/2 c of vegetable juice<br>1 c raw vegetables | Good source of vitamins and minerals, especially antioxidants; follow food safety guidelines in washing raw vegetables |
| Dairy | 8 oz (1 c) milk or yogurt<br>1-1/2 oz cheese<br>1-1/2 c frozen yogurt/ice cream | Good source of protein, B vitamins, and minerals; use pasteurized products |
| Protein foods | 3 oz cooked meat, chicken, or fish<br>2 cooked eggs<br>1/2 c nuts or tofu<br>1 c cooked dried beans, lentils, peas | Best sources of protein; good sources of B vitamins and minerals; 3 oz of meat is about the size of a deck of cards |

## Measuring Outcomes of Medical Nutrition Therapy

According to the HIV/AIDS MNT Protocol, one measurement of outcome is obtained by assessing the change in the patient's weight and LBM (4). In one study, the intervention, which was carried out by a dietitian, consisted of a nutritional status assessment, an individualized care plan, counseling, follow-up, and nutritional supplements as needed. Those in the intervention group had a median weight gain of 3 lb, whereas the nonintervention patients had a median loss of 4 lb (13). In another study, 56 inner-city patients with multiple risk factors were assessed nutritionally, clinically, and immunologically. The researchers concluded that subjects who had lost weight had a significantly lower BMI, decreased fat stores, reduced muscle mass, and lower CD4 cell counts than did subjects whose weight remained stable (40).

Other ways to measure the outcome of medical nutrition therapy are to check the change in the patient's food intake record over time, observe the trend in laboratory values, and evaluate the patient's response to medications, including nutritional side effects. Expected nutrition-related outcomes for the patient with HIV include the following (4):

- Meets goals set with dietitian.
- Takes steps to alleviate HIV-related symptoms.
- Maintains adequate caloric and protein levels.
- Prevents food-borne and water-borne illnesses.
- Maintains and enhances weight and LBM.
- Understands potential food-drug interactions.
- Participates in resistance exercise three times a week.
- Stops or limits smoking and use of caffeine, alcohol, and recreational drugs.
- Maintains hydration.

## Summary

It is essential to screen and assess the nutritional status of patients with HIV and AIDS. If an initial screening for general risk factors indicates poor nutritional status, a thorough nutrition assessment is recommended. This includes an evaluation of anthropometric measurements, biochemical values, drug-nutrient interactions, clinical findings, and nutrient intake. An important part of the nutrition assessment is the patient's medical and social history. Patient education also stresses the role of exercise in rehabilitation. Finally, monitoring measurement outcomes is another part of comprehensive medical nutrition therapy.

*References*

1. Position of The American Dietetic Association and The Canadian Dietetic Association: nutrition intervention in the care of persons with human immunodeficiency virus infection. *J Am Diet Assoc.* 1994;94:1042-1045.
2. White JV, Ham RH, Lipschitz DA, Dwyer JT, Wellman NS. Consensus of the Nutrition Screening Initiative: risk factors on indicators of poor nutritional status in older Americans. *J Am Diet Assoc.* 1991;91:783-787.
3. Nutrition Screening Initiative. *Nutrition Interventions Manual for Professionals*

*Caring for Older Americans: Executive Summary.* Washington, DC: Nutrition Screening Initiative; 1992.
4. HIV/AIDS Medical Nutrition Therapy Protocol. *Medical Nutrition Therapy Across the Continuum of Care.* Chicago, Ill: American Dietetic Association; 1996.
5. The Chicago Dietetic Association and The South Suburban Dietetic Association. *Manual of Clinical Dietetics.* 5th ed. Chicago, Ill: American Dietetic Association; 1996.
6. Ho DD. Viral counts count in HIV infection. *Science.* 1996;272:1124-1125.
7. Mellors JW, Rinaldo CR, Gupta P, White RM, Todd JA, Kingsley LA. Prognosis in HIV-1 infection predicted by the quantity of virus in plasma. *Science.* 1996;272:1167-1170.
8. Kotler DP, Tierney AR, Wang J, Pierson RN. Magnitude of body cell mass depletion and the timing of death from wasting in AIDS. *Am J Clin Nutr.* 1989;50:444-447.
9. Kotler DP. Nutritional effects and support in the patients with AIDS. *J Nutr.* 1992;122:723-727.
10. Timbo BB, Tollefson L. Nutrition: a cofactor in HIV disease. *J Am Diet Assoc.* 1994;94:1018-1022.
11. Chlebowski RT, Grosvenor MB, Bernhard NH, Morales LS, Bulcavage LM. Nutritional status, gastrointestinal dysfunction, and survival in patients with AIDS. *Am J Gastroenterol.* 1989;84:1288-1293.
12. Vaghefi SB, Castellon-Vogel EA. Nutrition and AIDS: an introductory Chapter. In: Watson RR, ed. *Nutrition and AIDS.* Ann Arbor, Mich: CRC Press; 1994:1-16.
13. McKinley MJ, Goodman-Block J. Lesser ML, Salbe AD. Improved body weight status as a result of nutrition intervention in adult, HIV-positive outpatients. *J Am Diet Assoc.* 1994;94:1014-1017.
14. Chlebowski RT, Grosvenor M, Lillington L, Sayre J, Beall G. Dietary intake and counseling, weight maintenance, and the course of HIV infection. *J Am Diet Assoc.* 1995;95:655-660.
15. Bahl S. Body weight, illness, and death. In: Bahl S, Hickson JF Jr. *Nutritional Care for HIV-Positive Persons: A Manual for Individuals and Their Caregivers.* Ann Arbor, Mich: CRC Press; 1995:37-49.
16. Wheeler D, Muurahainen N, Elion R, Launer C, Gilbert C, Bartsch G. Change in body weight as a predictor of death and opportunistic complications (OC) in HIV by history of prior OC. *Int Conf AIDS.* 1996;11:332. Abstract TuB2383.
17. Beaudette T, ed. Nutritional aspects of AIDS and HIV infection. *Semin Nutr.* 1995;14:1-17.
18. *Health Care and HIV: Nutritional Guide for Providers and Clients.* Vienna, Va: Bureau of Primary Health Care, US Department of Health and Human Services; 1996.
19. Hopkins B. Assessment of nutritional status. In: Gottschlich MM, Matarese LE, Shronts EP, eds. *Nutrition Support Dietetics.* 2nd ed. Silver Spring, Md: American Society for Parenteral and Enteral Nutrition; 1993:15-71.
20. Stein TP. Effect of HIV on metabolism and the relationship to muscle and body protein content. In: Watson RR, ed. *Nutrition and AIDS.* Ann Arbor, Mich: CRC Press; 1994:167-188.
21. Bioelectrical impedance analysis conference: December 1994 proceedings. *Am J Clin Nutr.* 1996;64(3 suppl):387S-532S. Conference statement on National Institutes of Health Web site: http://consensus.nih.gov.
22. Sluys R, van der Ende M, Swart M, van den Berg J, Wilson J. Body composition in patients with acquired immunodeficiency syndrome: a validation study of bioelectric impedance analysis. *JPEN* 1993;17:404-406.
23. Risser J, Rabeneck L, Foote L, Klish W. A comparison of fat-free mass estimates in men infected with the human immunodeficiency virus. *JPEN* 1995;19:28-32.
24. Ott M, Fischer H, Polat H, Helm EB, Frenz M, Caspary WF, Lembcke B. Bioelectrical impedance analysis as a predictor of survival in patients with human immunodeficiency virus infection. *J Acquir Immune Defic Syndr Hum Retrovirol.* 1995;9:20-25.

25. Moore FD, Oleson KH, McMurrey JD. The body cell mass and its supporting environment. In FD Moore, ed. *Body Composition in Health and Disease*. Philadelphia, Pa: WB Saunders; 1993.
26. Hayes CR, Ropka ME, Sebring NG, Anderson RE. Recent food intake did not influence precision of body composition estimates by bioelectrical impedance analysis in men with HIV infection. *J Am Diet Assoc*. 1996;96:386-388.
27. Thomson C. Specialized nutrition support. In: Watson RR, ed. *Nutrition and AIDS*. Ann Arbor, Mich: CRC Press; 1994:201-213.
28. Fenton M, Bowman J: Watch what you put in your mouth. *Positive Living*. August 1996.
29. Singer P, Katz DP, Dillon L, Kirvela O, Lazarus T, Askanazi J. Nutritional aspects of the acquired immunodeficiency syndrome. *Am J Gastroenterol*. 1992;87:265-273.
30. Bahl S. Drug-induced nutritional complications and their management. In: Bahl S, Hickson JF Jr. *Nutritional Care for HIV-Positive Persons: A Manual for Individuals and Their Caregivers*. Ann Arbor, Mich: CRC Press; 1995:95-113.
31. Fauci AS. AIDS in 1996: Much accomplished, much to do. *JAMA*. 1996;276:155-156. Editorial.
32. Bartlett JA, ed. *Care and Management of Patients With HIV Infection*. Durham, NC: Glaxo Wellcome Inc; 1996.
33. Crocker KS. Gastrointestinal manifestations of the acquired immunodeficiency syndrome. *Nursing Clin N Am*. 1989;24:395-406.
34. Bahl S: Oral and esophageal complications: nutritional management. In: Bahl S, Hickson JF Jr. *Nutritional Care for HIV-Positive Persons: A Manual for Individuals and Their Caregivers*. Ann Arbor, Mich: CRC Press; 1995:73-93.
35. Kotler DP, Tierney AR, Altileo D, Wang J, Pierson RN. Body mass repletion during ganciclovir therapy of cytomegalovirus infections in patients with the acquired immunodeficiency syndrome. *Arch Intern Med*. 1989;149:901-905.
36. Flaskerud JH. AIDS and traditional food therapies. In: Watson RR, ed. *Nutrition and AIDS*. Ann Arbor, Mich: CRC Press; 1994:235-247.
37. McArdle W, Katch F, Katch V. *Essentials of Exercise Physiology*. Philadelphia, Pa: Lea & Febiger; 1994:377-381.
38. Spence DW, Galantino MLA, Mossberg KA, Zimmerman SO. Progressive resistance exercise: effect on muscle function and anthropometry of a select AIDS population. *Arch Phys Med Rehab*. 1990;71:644-648.
39. Gibson RS. *Principles of Nutrition Assessment*. New York, NY: Oxford University Press; 1990.
40. Luder E, Godfrey E, Godbold J, Simpson DM. Assessment of nutritional, clinical, and immunologic status of HIV-infected, inner-city patients with multiple risk factors. *J Am Diet Assoc*. 1995;95:655-660.

# 3
# Oral Nutrition Interventions

Malnutrition and wasting are important cofactors in the human immunodeficiency virus (HIV) disease and the acquired immunodeficiency syndrome (AIDS). Their prevalence is such that nutrition education, individualized counseling, and oral nutrition intervention are essential in the early stages of the disease to enhance a patient's response to medications and other therapies, support immune function, and help prevent opportunistic infections and other signs of disease progression. Every effort must be made to encourage healthy eating in individuals with HIV. Long-term consequences of poor nutritional intake can include diminished quality of life, increased morbidity, and shortened life expectancy.

The causes of malnutrition are multifactorial and may include anorexia, gastrointestinal (GI) problems, food-drug interactions, and metabolic changes such as abnormal lipid metabolism and hypermetabolism (1, 2). Decreased body cell mass (BCM) and serum albumin and transferrin levels have been observed at every stage of HIV infection. Unless these factors are reversed, nutrition support alone may not be enough to treat malnutrition (3, 4). The nutrition care plan should include strategies to maintain and restore hydration, desirable body weight, and BCM and to provide adequate amounts of nutrients (5).

Decreased nutrient intake may be the primary concern for early nutrition interventions. Factors that affect a patient's appetite, weight, BCM, and ultimately survival are the focus of this chapter, along with guidelines for managing HIV symptoms that have dietary relevance. Vitamin and mineral supplementation is explored, followed by a section on oral nutritional supplements. Because many patients have questions about the benefits and risks of alternative therapies for HIV infection, this controversial subject is included here as well. And no matter what the topic for nutrition education, all counseling should be client-centered. Therefore, a section on nutrition counseling skills is included.

The nutrition needs of HIV-infected women during pregnancy and lactation are covered in the last section. The nutritional requirements of children are equally important. However, because the nutrition management of HIV problems in infants and children is unique and deserves detailed coverage, it will not be discussed in this book. The reader is referred for further information on this subject to references 16 and 38.

## Guidelines for Healthy Eating
### BASIC NUTRITION CARE FOR HIV-INFECTED PATIENTS

Because HIV disease is chronic, the need to know sound nutrition principles is great. The dietitian can play an important role in this area by educating the patient about adequate nutrition to maintain good nutritional status and healthful eating habits (5). Other important issues in nutrition education for patients with HIV include food safety guidelines, managing nutrition-related symptoms, and evaluation of alternative or complementary therapies (6). Nutrition education programs designed in accordance with existing beliefs of individual patients and their caretakers have a better chance of being accepted (7). For instance, if a patient has made a decision to become vegetarian, the dietitian can provide the necessary education to ensure optimal nutrient intake. Dietitians can network in person and on-line to discuss individual patient success stories and develop strategies to support nutritional intake and health (8).

The dietitian should take a careful nutrition history of each patient and assess usual food intake, paying special attention to fluids, kilocalories, and protein. With any reported problems or dietary restrictions, evaluation of fat, fiber, lactose, and other dietary components may come into play. Additional questions may include the use of vitamin and mineral supplements, herbal preparations, alcohol and recreational drugs, tobacco, over-the-counter medications, and caffeinated foods and beverages as appropriate. These and other questions are included in the HIV/AIDS Medical Nutrition Therapy (MNT) protocol (5). The patient should be advised to keep a food record (Figure 3-1) before a visit with the dietitian so that an individualized eating plan can be developed and eating problems can be pinpointed.

Oral feeding is preferred, provided that the GI tract is functional and the patient adequately tolerates food. If medical complications prevent an adequate intake and the patient is at risk for weight loss, enteral and even parenteral nutrition therapies (when the GI tract is no longer adequately functional) may be warranted (see Chapter 4).

### FOOD SAFETY

Food safety is of utmost importance to persons with HIV, whose immune systems are compromised and who are thus susceptible to food-borne illness from eating undercooked or poorly prepared foods. Food-borne illness or food poisoning can cause diarrhea, nausea, and vomiting, all of which can lead to weight loss. Inadequate access to resources and chronic fatigue, which results in limited energy to clean or

## FIGURE 3-1  Patient's Self-Monitoring Form for Food Intake

Name: _____  Date: _____

*Instructions*: Use this worksheet to evaluate your food intake. Fill this form out _____ days each week. Bring these worksheets with you to your next dietitian appointment on _____.

Date: _____                    Day of Week:  Sun   Mon   Tue   Wed   Thu   Fri   Sat

Food Group:                          Goal: _____ servings (minimum 3)
Meat, poultry, fish, eggs,           2-3 oz meats, 2 cooked eggs, 4 T peanut butter, 1 c
  dried beans, peas, nuts, seeds       cooked dried beans, 1/2 c nuts and seeds, 5-6 oz tofu
Minimum:                             Additional servings:


Food Group:                          Goal: _____ servings (minimum 3)
Milk, yogurt, cheese                 1 c milk, yogurt, ice cream, frozen yogurt, 1/2 c cottage cheese,
                                       1-2 oz cheese
Minimum:                             Additional servings:


Food Group:                          Goal: _____ servings (minimum 8-11)
Bread, cereal, rice, pasta           1 slice bread; 1/2 English muffin, bagel, or bun; 1 c flake-type cereal,
                                       1/2 c cooked cereal, rice, or pasta; 2 flour or corn tortillas, 6 saltine-
                                       type crackers, 3 squares graham crackers
Minimum:                             Additional servings:


Food Group:                          Goal: _____ servings (minimum 3)
Fruits                               1 medium-sized fruit (washed well); 1/2 c chopped, cooked, or canned
                                       fruit; 3/4 c fruit juice; 1/4 c dried fruit
Minimum:                             Additional servings:


Food Group:                          Goal: _____ servings (minimum 4)
Vegetables                           1 c leafy vegetables (washed well); 1/2 c cooked vegetables;
                                       3/4 c vegetable juice (carrot, tomato)
Minimum:                             Additional servings:


Fats and sweets (list):


Supplements (list):


Adverse symptoms or intolerances to specific foods (list):

shop for fresh groceries, may also promote unsanitary living conditions.

The following are guidelines for immunocompromised patients to follow in the kitchen:

- Drink sterilized water and avoid inadequately filtered tap water to avoid cryptosporidiosis and microsporidiosis (parasitic illnesses that can cause severe stomach cramps and diarrhea) and possible infection by *Mycobacterium avium-intracellulare*, which causes serious systemic disease in patients with AIDS. The Centers for Disease Control and Prevention (CDC) recommends boiling water for 1 minute to disinfect it for immunocompromised patients. Patients may also use filtration systems that can document adequate filtration for *Cryptosporidium* organisms.
- Check expiration dates on foods in the grocery store and in the pantry to make sure they are current.
- Keep hot foods hot and cold foods cold. Bacteria in food multiplies the most at room temperature. The danger zone for temperature is between 40 and 140°F.
- "If in doubt, throw it out." Because foods containing harmful bacteria do not always look or smell bad, do not ingest foods past their expiration date. See Table 3-1 for storage time limits for various refrigerated and frozen products.
- Wash hands with warm, soapy water and rinse well before and after preparation of foods.
- Thoroughly clean and brush all fruits and vegetables with water and mild soap or lemon juice. Or remove the skin or peel before eating fruits and vegetables.
- Avoid eating raw or undercooked meat or fish.

### TABLE 3-1 Storage Limits for Refrigerated and Frozen Foods

| Product | Use Within | Product | Use Within |
|---|---|---|---|
| **Refrigerated foods (stored at 35-40°F)** | | Fresh eggs in the shell | 3 wk |
| Raw beefsteaks and roasts, raw pork chops, raw lamb chops and roasts, cooked ham, lunch meat | 3-5 d | Raw yolks or whites (out of the shell) | 2-4 d |
|  |  | Hard-cooked eggs | 7 d |
| Ground beef, turkey, pork, or lamb; sausage | 1-2 d | **Frozen foods** | |
|  |  | Bread | 24 mo |
| Hot dogs | 7 d | Bacon | 3 mo |
| Raw chicken or turkey; giblets | 1-2 d | Cooked dishes (roast meats, casseroles) | 1-3 mo |
| Leftover cooked meat and meat dishes; soups and stews | 3-4 d | Fresh fruit | 8-12 mo |
|  |  | Fish/shellfish | 4-6 mo/2-3 mo |
| Leftover gravy and meat broth | 1-2 d | Meat, poultry, rabbit, game | 8-10 mo |
| Leftover cooked poultry and poultry dishes | 3-4 d | Pastry (raw dough) | 3 mo |
| Leftover cooked poultry covered with broth or gravy; leftover chicken nuggets, patties, or fried chicken | 1-2 d | Vegetables | 6-9 mo |

Sources: Labuza TP, Erdman JW. *Food Science and Nutritional Health: An Introduction.* St Paul, Minn: West Publishing; 1984; Harvey J, ed. *Larousse Gastronomique: The New American Edition of the World's Greatest Culinary Encyclopedia.* New York, NY: Crown Publishers; 1984; Salomon SB, Davis M, Fields-Gardner C: *Living Well with HIV and AIDS: A Guide to Healthy Eating.* Chicago, Ill: American Dietetic Association; 1993.

- Avoid thawing frozen poultry and meat at room temperature. Use a microwave or thaw in a refrigerator instead.
- Discard leftovers that have been in the refrigerator for more than 3 days.
- Do not buy unpasteurized dairy products; they may contain *Salmonella* organisms.
- Avoid eating eggs with cracked shells. Avoid undercooked eggs that are scrambled but runny, soft-boiled, or sunny-side up. Do not eat foods that contain raw eggs, such as cookie or cake batter, homemade mayonnaise and eggnog, Caesar salad dressing, chocolate mousse, and some frostings (3, 9, 10).

## HIGH-ENERGY AND HIGH-PROTEIN FOOD CHOICES

Because persons with HIV tend to be hypermetabolic, and an infection or malignancy places additional energy and protein demands on the body, a high-protein, high-energy diet is often recommended (11,12). Some patients may require up to 45 to 50 kcal/kg/day (3). Basal energy expenditure (BEE) in HIV-positive patients may be calculated using the Harris-Benedict formula and then adjusting it by adding increases for activity, metabolic stress, and requirements to maintain or gain weight. In severe infection, adjustment can range from 1.4 to 1.8 times BEE (3,13). Often the best way to determine energy needs is to monitor energy intake over time to determine at what level the patient maintains or is able to gain weight. To maintain body protein stores, higher levels than normal (0.8 g/kg body weight) may be required at approximately 1 to 1.4 g protein per kg body weight. Repletion and anabolic strategies may require 1.5-2.0 g protein per kg body weight (3).

The following strategies can help patients incorporate more calories and protein into their diets. Note that strategies should be individualized according to patients' preferences and tolerances.

- Eat more small meals, as many as six to nine, spaced throughout the day.
- Emphasize complex carbohydrate foods such as whole-grain breads and cereals, pasta, potatoes, rice, and corn.
- Add calories with quick snacks such as dried fruit and cookies. Serve jelly, honey, and maple syrup for breakfast. Add sugar to tea and milk shakes.
- If fat is tolerated, have a peanut butter sandwich for lunch or add butter or margarine to peas, potatoes, and other vegetables. Add nuts to salads, cooked vegetables, and casseroles. Other high-fat items include bacon, sour cream, cream cheese, olives, gravy, avocado, and salad dressings.
- Eat generous amounts of food-based protein at each meal, from either animal or vegetable sources. Add diced chicken, tofu cubes, and cooked beans to soups and salads. Use grated cheese in sauces, soups, omelets, and salads. Enjoy yogurt milkshakes. Add dry, powdered milk to soups, gravies, milk shakes, and hot cereals. Monitor tolerance of these dairy products (10).

It may be necessary to spend time convincing the patient that these types of foods are preferable when energy and protein intake is jeopardized. As target energy and protein levels are reached, alternate strategies for lower fat foods may be counseled.

## Common Dietary Problems

### ANOREXIA

Anorexia is a primary barrier to adequate oral intake of nutrients in HIV-infected persons. A loss of appetite may be caused by depression, medications, weakness and fatigue, fever, HIV-related dementia, and the body's stress response to infections. Because minimizing weight loss and preserving BCM are desirable outcomes, the following dietary recommendations have been formulated to combat decreased oral intake due to anorexia and to stimulate the patient's appetite:

- Eat small, frequent meals and follow a regular schedule for meals; that is, "eat by the clock."
- Avoid stress, such as family arguments, at mealtimes and immediately before meals.
- Select favorite foods, keeping some within easy reach (near the bed or couch).
- Avoid foods with a strong odor.
- Do light exercises recommended by a physician or physical therapist to increase your appetite (3, 10).

One way to cope with low food intake caused by fatigue is to keep the freezer stocked with single portions from foods made in advance when the patient feels energetic enough to cook. If the patient cannot cook or is too weak to do so, the dietitian can arrange for or refer the patient to homemaker services through a social service agency or can arrange for home-delivered meals. (See Chapter 5 and Appendix D for community-based nutrition resources in HIV and AIDS care.)

Overcoming anorexia may require a pharmacologic approach. Megestrol acetate (Megace, Bristol Myers Squibb Co, Princeton, NJ 08543) has been studied the most in patients with AIDS. Derived from progesterone, a steroid used as chemotherapy to treat breast cancer, megestrol has been shown to be beneficial in stimulating appetite. In comparing megestrol acetate with a placebo, Van Roenn et al (14) found that a dose of 800 mg/day improved weight gain and mood more than the placebo among 270 patients with AIDS. Tested in 10 HIV-infected men, megestrol therapy resulted in increased appetite in all subjects and weight gain in eight of the 10 patients (15). Another medical report focused on seven HIV-infected children and adolescents, aged 26 months to 20 years, who not only gained weight while receiving megestrol but also were more active and less tired (16). Drawbacks to megestrol are its cost, up to approximately $7,000 per year but $3,200 for the generic product (17), and weight gains primarily in the adipose tissue rather than in lean body mass (16, 18). Other drawbacks include impotence, vaginal spotting (19), and adrenal insufficiency (20). However, therapy may be worth the expense when it vastly improves a patient's overall nutritional status and therefore quality of life.

Dronabinol (Marinol, Roxane Laboratories, Columbus, OH 43228) is another pharmacologic agent tested in HIV-seropositive persons. Derived from *Cannabis sativa* (marijuana) (21), dronabinol is used to control nausea in cancer patients undergoing chemotherapy. In two studies involving HIV-infected persons (22, 23), dronabinol stimulated the appetite in 33 of 35 patients. The lowest dose (2.5 mg twice daily) was tolerated best; however, unpleasant side effects associated with this drug included drowsiness, confusion, impaired coordination, anxiety, and lack of concentration. Beal et al (24) found in 1995 that dronabinol was safe and effective for patients with AIDS and that side effects ranged from mild to moderate in severity. They concluded that dronabinol was associated with increased appetite, improved mood, reduced nausea, and stabilized weight.

Other agents that stimulate appetite include cyproheptadine (Periactin, Merck & Co, West Point, PA 19486), hydrazine sulfate, and corticosteroids. In the last category, prednisone, at a dose of 10 mg/day, was found to be as effective as megestrol in increasing appetite and weight gain and, moreover, is less expensive (about $5 per month) (25). However, the disadvantages of corticosteroids, such as immunosuppression, muscle weakness, electrolyte imbalance, hyperglycemia, and fluid retention, preclude their long-term use. Furthermore, the effect of appetite enhancement disappears after a few weeks (19). These agents can be used as a last resort when low testosterone levels prevent the use of megestrol. Some of these agents are contraindicated in patients using certain protease inhibitor therapies. The clinicians should check current company guidelines if corticosteroids are being considered.

## NAUSEA AND VOMITING

Infection, GI illness, cancer, inadequate pain control, and some medications may contribute to nausea and vomiting. Effective interventions for patients include the following:

- Avoid dehydration by replacing fluids and electrolytes.
- Drink beverages between meals rather than with meals.
- Eat slowly.
- Do not lie down right after eating.
- Serve small, frequent meals.
- Choose cold foods, such as a roast beef sandwich.
- Try dry, salty, and bland foods such as toast or crackers.
- Avoid foods with strong odors.
- Use antiemetic drugs.
- If a certain medicine is causing nausea, ask your physician or pharmacist for advice about taking it at a different time (3,10).

## MOUTH PAIN AND SWALLOWING DIFFICULTIES

Many complications of HIV disease, such as oral and esophageal lesions, malignant tumors that cause mouth pain and burning or throat obstruction, neurologic disorders, and side effects of medicines, make chewing and swallowing difficult. Proper medical and dental care are important to treat and lessen these conditions. If the patient has mouth pain or sores, the following guidelines may be helpful:

- Avoid smoking, alcohol, and carbonated sodas, which can be irritants to mouth sores.
- Let hot foods cool before eating to avoid burning oral tissues.
- Ice-cold foods such as sherbet, sorbet, ice cream, frozen yogurt, and other frozen treats can help numb soreness.
- If the patient has oral ulcers, a soft diet is recommended. Soft, bland foods that are soothing include applesauce, oatmeal, cottage cheese, custards and puddings, creamy soups, and hard-boiled eggs.
- Frequent use of mouth rinses may relieve sore gums.

Antidotes for patients who suffer painful swallowing include:

- Opt for soft or pureed foods or foods prepared in a blender.
- Use a straw when drinking beverages.
- Tilt your head back while swallowing.
- Drink soup out of a mug.
- Avoid foods that are too hot or too cold; wait until they have reached room temperature (3,10).

If the patient's condition warrants extra energy and protein, an easy-to-swallow nutritional supplement may be in order (see Table 3-2 and the section "Oral Nutritional Supplements").

## TASTE ALTERATIONS (DYSGEUSIA)

The sense of taste can be affected by infections and medications. Bad tastes can range from metallic to garlicky. When patients have a bitter, metallic taste in their mouths, bland food may help, and so may the following:

- Eat with plastic utensils.
- Prepare a soothing daily mouth rinse to prevent thrush by mixing 1 tsp baking soda with a glass of warm, distilled water. Do not swallow the mixture; swallowing a baking soda solution may cause mild stomach upset in some patients.
- Mask the metallic taste by drinking tart beverages (lemonade, orange juice, and cranberry juice) and by adding acidic condiments (vinegar, lemon juice, pickles, and relish) to foods.
- Marinate meat, fowl, fish, and tofu in wine, vinegar, salad dressing, or soy sauce to avoid a metallic taste.
- Use seasonings such as rosemary, thyme, basil, oregano, and cumin.
- Vary the textures of food from hard and crisp to soft and smooth to add interest and variety to eating.
- To numb the metallic taste, select cold foods such as sherbet, fruit ice, ice cream, sorbet, and frozen yogurt.
- To stimulate saliva, try sour sugarless candy and cold foods.
- Ask about mouth-coating artificial saliva products (10).

**TABLE 3-2  Oral Nutrition Supplements**

| Formula Manufacturer[a] | Description of Selected Contents |
|---|---|
| Advera (Ross) | Peptides, fiber, additional micronutrients (eg, beta carotene), n-3 fatty acids—fish oil; vanilla and chocolate in ready-to-use (RTU) creamy liquid |
| AlitraQ (Ross) | Hydrolyzed protein, glutamine, arginine, medium-chain triglycerides (MCT), low-fat flavor packets in clear powder |
| BeneFit (Hoechst Marion Rousel) | Intact nutrients, fiber available; vanilla and chocolate creamy liquid; bars |
| Citrisource (Novartis) | Protein supplement (egg white base) with vitamins and minerals; fruit-flavored RTU clear liquid |
| Ensure (Ross) | Intact protein, fiber available; many flavors in RTU creamy liquid |
| HealthGain (Metagenics) | Hydrolyzed lactalbumin; low-fat vanilla, chocolate, and orange flavors in creamy powder |
| Immun-Aid (McGaw) | Lactalbumin, arginine, glutamine, branded-chain amino acids (BCAA), MCT; lemon-lime and orange flavors in clear powder |
| Lipisorb (Mead Johnson) | Intact protein, MCT; vanilla RTU creamy liquid and powder |
| Magnacal (Sherwood Medical) | Intact protein, high calorie (2 kcal/mL); vanilla RTU creamy liquid |
| NuBasics (Nestle) | Intact protein, MCT; 1, 1.5, and 2 kcal/mL; variety of flavors in RTU creamy liquid; bars; coffee; soups |
| Peptamen (Nestle) | Hydrolyzed protein, MCT; RTU clear liquid, flavor packets |
| Resource, Resource Plus (Novartis) | Intact nutrients; Resource Plus is higher protein; variety of flavors in RTU creamy liquid and powder |
| ScandiShake (Scandipharm) | Calorie dense (600 kcal/with 8 oz whole milk), MCT; lactose-free and sugar-free available; not complete nutrition; vanilla, strawberry, and chocolate creamy powder; taste-free powder |
| Sustacal (Mead Johnson) | Intact protein, 20% fat; variety of flavors in RTU creamy liquid and powder |
| Vivonex Plus (Novartis) | Amino acids; very low-fat flavor packets, powder |

Manufacturer information: Ross Products Division, Abbott Laboratories, Abbott Park, IL 60064; Hoechst Marion Rousel, Kansas City, MO 64134; Novartis Nutrition, Fremont, MI 47413; Metagenics, San Clemente, CA 92673; McGaw, Irvine, CA 92714; Mead Johnson Nutritionals, Evansville, IN 47721; Sherwood Medical, St. Louis, MO 63103; Nestle Clinical Information, Deerfield, IL 60015; and Scandipharm, Inc, Birmingham, AL 35242.

## XEROSTOMIA

Xerostomia, a disorder characterized by a dry mouth, can be managed by using artificial saliva and sugarless lemon drops (26). A liquid diet and moist foods, such as gravies, sauces, yogurt, and puddings, are also helpful. Adequate fluid intake is essential (see Chapter 4 for calculating fluid requirements). For many patients, this may mean drinking at least 2 qt (1.136 L) of fluids a day.

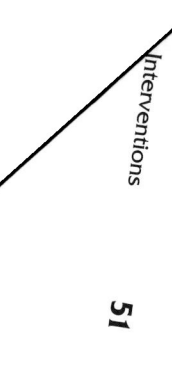

## DIARRHEA AND CONSTIPATION

Medications may be the culprit behind diarrhea, but so could an infection of the GI tract or GI surgery. There are four types of diarrhea: osmotic, secretory, exudative, and limited mucosal contact (Table 3-3). The first principle of diarrhea management is to identify and treat the cause of the diarrhea. However, symptomatic management should be used concurrently. Rehydration and electrolyte replacement may need to be done parenterally in cases of copious diarrhea. Parenteral nutrition should be considered if adequate oral intake is not anticipated within a few days.

Depending on the cause of the diarrhea, here are some dietary methods that can help patients cope with this problem:

- Avoid caffeine and alcohol.
- Avoid high-fat foods such as bacon, sausage, and cold cuts, especially if malabsorption is causing the diarrhea due to various intestinal infections or medication interactions. Eat soft cooked fish, chicken, turkey, or lean beef.
- If lactose intolerance is a problem, avoid milk and use a low-lactose or lactose-free diet. Lactase-supplemented milk (Lactaid, McNeil-PPC Inc, Fort Washington, PA 19034) or low-fat soy milk may be substituted for lactose-intolerant individuals and for others during periods of diarrhea. Gradually reincorporate milk products as diarrhea subsides, if possible.
- Drink plenty of fluids at room temperature, especially those that contain calories: lemonade, sports drinks, punch, and juices (except for apple juice).
- Avoid certain high-fiber foods containing cellulose fiber, such as fruits (except for bananas and applesauce), vegetables, whole grains, and corn. Consider canned fruits and vegetables or well-cooked vegetables as tolerated.
- Try high-soluble fiber foods such as oatmeal, white rice, barley, and pureed vegetables and fruits (eg, applesauce).

**TABLE 3-3 Symptomatic Management of Diarrhea**

| Type | Characteristics | Recommendations |
| --- | --- | --- |
| Osmotic | Presence of poorly absorbed osmotically active solutes | Reduce osmotic load, feed isotonic formulations |
| Secretory | Secretion of electrolytes and water by intestinal epithelium; not relieved by fasting | General diarrhea control recommendations; may require bowel rest and/or parenteral nutrition |
| Exudative | Mucus, blood, and plasma protein losses associated with mucosal damage (eg, chronic ulcerative colitis and radiation enteritis) | Monitor carefully for multiple nutrient deficiencies; replace protein, fluid, and other nutrient loss; may require bowel rest and/or parenteral nutrition |
| Limited mucosal contact | Reduced bile salt concentration and/or steatorrhea, resulting from inadequate exposure of chyme to intestinal wall | Low-fat or alternate fat source may be indicated; soluble fibers; parenteral fluid or nutrient replacement; antimotility medication |

- Do not eat foods associated with cramping or bloating. These appear to be highly individual and may include foods such as cabbage, beans, broccoli, brussels sprouts, onions, radishes, and green peppers.
- Select high-potassium foods and beverages, such as bananas, potatoes, sports drinks, diluted orange juices, and fruit nectars to replace stores lost in diarrhea.

Dehydration can be a major problem in HIV-infected patients, sometimes necessitating hospitalization and immediate intravenous (IV) fluids. The signs and symptoms of dehydration include decreased skin turgor, lethargy, dry oral membranes, decreased urine output, increased hematocrit, and/or weight loss greater than 1% per day (3). More severe signs of dehydration include rapid, thready pulse, increased blood pressure, rapid breathing, and decreased level of consciousness (3). Severe diarrhea can lead to a loss of fluid and electrolytes (sodium, potassium, magnesium, and chloride). Parenteral fluids with electrolytes are necessary for patients in shock or who are severely dehydrated with fluid deficits of 10% or more.

Some patients may complain of constipation. In this case, enhance their intake of foods that may shorten transit time. This can include a variety of whole grain breads and cereals; oatmeal cookies; fig, date, or raisin bars; granola bars; and fruits and vegetables. Intermittent use of bulking agents (eg, Metamucil, Procter & Gamble, Cincinnati, OH 45201) with plenty of fluids may help relieve constipation. Light exercise such as walking may also help. Cathartic efforts such as prune juice or laxative medications may be recommended on occasion as needed.

## Vitamin and Mineral Supplementation

Because alterations in vitamins A, E, B-6, and B-12; riboflavin; copper; zinc; and selenium have been found in persons with HIV infection, some patients may need supplementation (3). Research studies have found mixed results. In one study involving 296 HIV-infected men, intakes of iron, vitamin E, and riboflavin (all exceeding 200% of the RDA) were significantly associated with delayed development of AIDS (27). Abrams et al (27) therefore suggested that the use of multivitamin-mineral supplements may have a role in maintaining an asymptomatic stage. In another study, 21 patients in various stages of HIV infection received beta carotene supplements (180 mg/day), which transiently increased the total white blood cell (WBC) count, CD4 cell count, and CD4-to-CD8 ratio (1).

Tang et al (28) discussed delayed progression to a diagnosis of AIDS with greater intakes of thiamin, niacin, and vitamin C. Results of this same study suggested that the highest intakes of vitamin A and zinc may be related somehow to a more rapid progression to an AIDS-defining complication.

In 1997 Tang et al (29) reported on the association between serum vitamin A and E levels and HIV-1 disease progression in 311 HIV-seropositive homosexual or bisexual men participating in the Multicenter AIDS Cohort Study. They found that elevated serum vitamin E levels were associated with a decreased risk of progression to AIDS and mortality. This association, however, was not found in vitamin A. These results suggest that support for higher serum vitamin E levels should be further explored for potential benefits in delaying the onset of AIDS in HIV-1-infected persons.

Although these studies do not provide clear evidence for supplementation of nutrients, they open the question for further exploration. Obviously, more studies are needed to confirm the association between micronutrient supplements and HIV disease progression. In the meantime, many physicians and dietitians are recommending a balanced multivitamin and mineral supplement at levels of approximately 100% of the US RDA (8). Single vitamin and mineral supplementation should be monitored by the HIV health care team. Individual nutrients taken in excess can accumulate in the body and cause problems, such as diarrhea, nausea, and anorexia, as well as damage or alter organ function. It is important for the patient to know that even a balanced multivitamin and mineral supplement does not replace healthful food choices and eating patterns. See Figure 3-2 for a worksheet to evaluate a patient's intake of supplements.

Supplementation is an effort to augment antioxidant activity in the cells. Whether exogenous sources of antioxidants and their precursors have the ability to enhance the endogenous supply remains to be elucidated. Some clinicians have recommended a series of antioxidant supplements, such as glutathione, *N*-acetylcysteine, vitamins C and E, and beta carotene. Antioxidants from food have the potential not only to be balanced but also to work synergistically (and possibly more powerfully) with other food substances, such as flavonoids and pigments, that also contain antioxidants (30, 31).

## Oral Nutritional Supplements

When a patient does not feel hungry or is not tolerating a general diet, a commercially prepared nutritional supplement is an option (see Table 3-2). Standard supplements (eg, Ensure, Ross Products Division, Abbott Laboratories, Abbott Park, IL 60064; Resource, Novartis Nutrition, Fremont, MI 47413, and Sustacal, Mead Johnson Nutritionals, Evansville, IN 47721) contain intact nutrients and vitamins and minerals to provide complete nutrition care. A fully functioning GI tract is necessary to tolerate these supplements, as some patients may have problems with fat malabsorption or diarrhea with intact formulas.

If lactose intolerance is not a problem, a breakfast drink (Carnation Instant Breakfast) is an inexpensive alternative to nutrition supplements; if lactose intolerance is a concern, a breakfast drink can be used in combination with a lactase supplement or with lactase-supplemented milk or soy milk (31, 33). Scandishake (Scandipharm Inc, Birmingham, AL 35242) is also an inexpensive source of kilocalories (600 kcal per 8-oz serving) and offers lactose-free and aspartame-sweetened counterparts.

The unpleasant taste of supplements is a common complaint of many HIV-infected patients. Decaffeinated coffee powder, uncarbonated

## FIGURE 3-2  Sample Worksheet for Supplements

Patient Name/Chart Number: _____  Date: _____

| Intake analysis: | ❑ 24-hour recall | ❑ typical day recall | ❑ averaged food diary ( _____ day) |
| Analysis by: | ❑ computer | ❑ exchange lists | ❑ other:_____ |

Estimated requirements
or goals:                            Intake analysis:                 Deficit:                         Excess:

*Macronutrients:*

Fluids: _____

Kilocalories:_____

Protein: _____

Carbohydrates: _____

Fat: _____

*Micronutrients:*

*Other:* (eg, fiber)

Food Recommendations:                                     Supplement Recommendations:

---

soft drinks, gelatin powder, or commercial flavor packets may improve their taste.

Predigested elemental lactose-free formulas may be more appropriate to give the GI tract a rest if lactose intolerance and GI tract dysfunction are problems. Diarrhea or malabsorption may be helped by a low-fat supplement, such as Sustacal or one with MCT oil (Lipisorb, Mead Johnson Nutritionals; Nutren and Peptamen, Nestle), in which the fat is more easily digested and absorbed (34). Sometimes higher fat supplements may be used in conjunction with enteric-coated pancreatic lipase.

If the diarrhea is severe, the patient may need a predigested or partially digested formula (Vivonex Plus, Novartis; Criticare, Mead Johnson; Peptamen, Nestle; and Impact, Novartis). Supplements such as Peptamen and Reabilan provide an increased amount of protein in the form of peptides. Vivonex Plus is an example of a free amino acid based formula. In addition, there are HIV-specific formulas (Advera, Ross Products Division, Abbott Laboratories, Abbott Park, IL 60064) which contain added n-3 fatty acids from fish oil, beta carotene, fiber, and peptides. More studies are needed in this area to help the dietitian decide on the most appropriate product to use in the various situations that challenge maintenance of nutritional status. Test different supplements until some are found that the patient can tolerate and is willing to drink.

## Alternative Therapies

According to Barrett (35), 54 of 79 patients visiting the St Louis AIDS Clinical Trials Unit had experimented with an alternative treatment, such as vitamins, herbs, and unapproved drugs. Additionally, 25 of 114 patients who attended the AIDS Clinic of the University of California-San Francisco Medical Center had tried an herbal product (35).

In evaluating whether a patient should or should not try an alternative therapy, the most important determining factor is whether the therapy has potential harmful side effects. If no risks are associated with the therapy and legitimate medical treatment is not being rejected, psychological benefits to the patient may outweigh any criticism that a clinician may have (3). See Table 3-4 for risks associated with alternative therapies (3, 35-39).

According to an American Medical Association publication (40), alternative methods have appeal because of the following:

- The methods are promoted extensively in the media and by word of mouth.
- Alternative treatment is viewed as painless and more natural, whereas conventional treatment is seen as often having toxic, chemical side effects.
- Patients may be disenchanted with conventional medicine and desperate for a cure.
- Proponents of alternative therapy use simple, everyday language such as "detoxification" and "buildup of toxins."
- Control over their lives is an important aspect as patients prepare special foods or take supplements and, hence, participate actively in their own therapy.
- Some patients use both conventional and complementary techniques to make certain that they cover all bases.

In addition, some of the complementary therapies may promise quick, dramatic, and even miraculous results (35). Dietitians who insist that HIV-infected clients conform only to the HIV/AIDS MNT protocol and not use alternative therapies may find that they have a low adherence rate (7). Trying to change a person's mind about HIV and its treatment in a few short sessions may be counterproductive. Therapeutic dietary regimens will be more effective if the client's dietary beliefs—those that are beneficial and neutral—are incorporated as much as possible. Just as dietitians use patient experiences and feedback when doing nutrition education and counseling, they should be open to the possible

## TABLE 3-4  Effects of Alternative Therapies for HIV Infection

| Therapy | Comments/Potential Side Effects |
| --- | --- |
| **Unlikely or Less Toxic Side Effects** | |
| Vitamin E | Least toxic of fat-soluble vitamins: up to 800 mg/d (36) |
| Beta carotene | Capable of modulating immune markers; effect is maximal after 3 months but diminished in 4th month; vitamin A can be toxic in megadoses |
| Artemisia (Qing Hao or QHS) | Antimicrobial; no reported side effects (3) |
| Blue-green algae (Spirulina) | Promoted for increasing immunity and boosting energy (35); no reported side effects (3) |
| Coenzyme $Q_{10}$ | Purported as an antioxidant and immune modulator (3) |
| **Potentially Toxic** | |
| Germanium-32 | Claimed to be an antioxidant and immunostimulatory (3) |
| Iron | A dose >20 times the Recommended Daily Allowances (RDA) for 6 wk impairs immune function; caution should be taken (36) |
| Zinc | A dose >20 times the RDA for 6 wk impairs immune function (36); prolonged daily intakes >2 g are toxic (39) |
| Acemannan (Carisyn) | Derived from the aloe vera plant; purported to be anti-HIV and immunostimulatory; nausea, vomiting, and abdominal pain (3) |
| Bitter melon (MAP-30) | Claimed to be an antiviral but toxic in long-term use |
| Compound Q (GLQ223) | A wide range of side effects from unpleasant (pain in muscles and joints, hives, and rashes) to dangerous and deadly (progression of Kaposi's sarcoma and coma) or death |
| Vitamin C | If taken in excess, can cause diarrhea, making it hazardous for HIV patients (37) |
| Glycyrrhizin | Touted as a cough and cold remedy; derived from licorice root; toxic effects from excessive quantities include high blood pressure and cardiac problems |
| Hypericin | Purported antiviral; derived from Saint-John's-wort; photosensitivity is the side effect (38) |
| Selenium | Highly toxic; may suppress immune function at >200 µg/d and damage the liver and nervous system |

Sources: The Chicago Dietetic Association and The South Suburban Dietetic Association (reference 3); Barret S (35); Vaghefi SB, Castellon-Vogel EA (36); Herbert V (37); Tyler VE (38); and Dwyer JT, Bye RL, Holt PL, Lauze SR (39).

benefits of alternate therapies, even if traditional double-blind, placebo-controlled studies have not been completed.

## Nutrition Counseling Skills

Optimally, the dietitian and an HIV-infected client will establish a trusting and cooperative working relationship. The dietitian's careful listening, empathy, and response to the patient's needs can make the difference between effective and ineffective nutrition care. By conducting interviews in a nonjudgmental style, the dietitian will elicit more accurate responses from the patient and build a strong patient-clinician rapport. Confidentiality and other standards of professional conduct cannot be emphasized enough. For instance, it is inappropriate to request information on how the virus was contracted (mode of transmission), when the purpose of the visit is to provide nutrition counseling. The clinician must make sure the consent to release medical information is in place and that confidentiality is completely respected.

Keep in mind that patients may be frightened, shocked, or depressed in their efforts to cope with this chronic disease. A feeling that HIV infection controls one's life is not uncommon among patients. The dietitian can help the patient feel more in control by first determining his or her wants and needs during each counseling session and, together, setting mutual goals. Examples of goals include the following: maintain or replenish weight and muscle mass, control nutrition-related symptoms, improve the quality of life, and other outcomes mentioned previously.

Change is difficult, even under the best circumstances, and living with HIV is stressful. Suggest one change at a time, and make certain that your recommendations are realistic (10). In client-centered nutrition counseling, dos and don'ts have given way to the client making a choice among various options (41). Setting priorities for recommendations, explaining nutrition assessment measures, and providing practical suggestions, including giving menus, recipes, and guidelines to manage symptoms such as anorexia, diarrhea, nausea, vomiting, and weight loss, can enable patients to make their own decisions. By supporting decisions that can improve overall health status, the dietitian encourages the patient's sense of having control over his or her life.

Additional strategies for dietitians include the following: be an active listener, suspend judgment, be aware of body language, and help clients set priorities with nutrition goals (42, 43). It is important for dietitians to communicate nutrition information according to the patient's own cultural values and beliefs (7).

## Nutrition Needs of HIV-Infected Women During Pregnancy and Lactation

The problems of women with HIV infection have been eclipsed by their isolation, poverty, minority status, and lack of access to basic health services (44). Also, because of the social stigma associated with HIV infection and AIDS, some women and their families may be embarrassed to disclose the disease to health providers. For these reasons, the prevalence of HIV and AIDS in women and children may be underestimated (44).

As noted in Chapter 1, HIV is increasingly affecting women. In the United States, the number of women with AIDS rose 9% in just 1 year from 1994 to 1995, according to the CDC (45). Although more men than women were diagnosed with AIDS in the United States in 1995, the rate of increase for men was less (<1%) compared with 1994. Still, there are more men in the United States with AIDS compared with women (465,904 men vs 82,198 women), according to the CDC (46). Worldwide, 9.2 million women have HIV or AIDS and account for 42% of the total, but this proportion is increasing (47). These survey results highlight the need for targeted efforts by dietitians specializing in HIV and AIDS to reach women of childbearing age who are HIV positive. Of particular challenge are the special nutrition needs of women during pregnancy and lactation, which may compound the burden imposed by the HIV infection itself.

## PRENATAL CARE

When pregnancy and HIV infection occur together, there may be a negative synergetic effect on immune function. Both pregnancy and HIV infection impose physiological stresses on the body. Both affect the immune response in women, thereby increasing their vulnerability to viral, bacterial, and fungal infections (10). Both increase metabolism, which in turn increases the requirements for energy, protein, and micronutrients. Hence, these superimposed demands on the HIV-positive pregnant woman necessitate regular serial nutrition assessments and early nutrition intervention (44).

As discussed in Chapter 2, tools to assess nutritional status include anthropometric, biochemical, clinical, and dietary data. The dietitian specializing in HIV also needs to inquire about the patient's medical history, including outcomes of previous pregnancies, and psychosocial background, including the socioeconomic level, support of family and friends, and access to community nutrition services if necessary (see Chapter 5). Questions about use of alcohol, tobacco, and drugs of abuse are also pertinent. Input from a dietitian who specializes in perinatal nutrition and referral records from the patient's primary health care provider and/or obstetrician can be most valuable. Together, this information comprises important baseline data for developing an individualized nutrition care plan.

It is well established that the nutritional well-being of a healthy mother-to-be is crucial for an uncomplicated pregnancy and positive outcome. Prematurity, malnutrition, and low birth weight in the neonate are more common in HIV-infected mothers than in their healthy counterparts (44). Hence, healthful eating habits are indispensable in the HIV-infected pregnant woman. Early nutrition intervention can not only affect maternal and fetal health but also strengthen nutrition-related immunity.

Special nutritional requirements during pregnancy of HIV-positive women have not been documented (44). Start with established nutrition guidelines for a normal pregnancy: 300 additional kilocalories and 60 g of high-quality protein plus an appropriate, balanced vitamin or mineral supplement. Any additions to these estimated needs should be individualized. The patient should be assessed for other risk factors, such as adolescence, previously existing malnutrition, underweight status at the start of pregnancy, insufficient weight gain during pregnancy, iron-deficiency anemia, pregnancy-induced hypertension, gestational diabetes, and opportunistic infection. Even during a risk-free pregnancy, the need is high for extra vitamins and minerals such as the B vitamins, vitamin C, folic acid, calcium, and iron (10). Questions in HIV-complicated pregnancy that remain to be resolved in research include which nutrients are needed and in what amounts.

Prenatal care includes regularly monitoring the weight gain pattern throughout pregnancy. The National Academy of Sciences (NAS) recommends the following weight gains for healthy pregnant women: 25 to 35 lb for women of normal weight, 28 to 40 lb for underweight women, and 15 to 25 lb for overweight women (48). In general, energy requirements for HIV-positive or other pregnant women may range from 2,400 to 3,000 kcal (44). Barriers to gaining weight during an HIV-complicated pregnancy include diarrhea, nausea, vomiting, malabsorption, dysphagia, and opportunistic infections. Unexplained rapid weight loss in anyone, but especially in an HIV-positive mother-to-be, requires prompt medical attention and dietary intervention. If diarrhea and vomiting are severe, weight gain is inadequate, eating habits are poor, and oral supplements are not tolerated, enteral or parenteral support may be necessary (see Chapter 4).

## MOTHER-TO-CHILD TRANSMISSION OF HIV

Not every pregnant woman with AIDS transmits HIV to her infant. Still, it is estimated that there is a 15% to 45% risk that the virus will be transmitted perinatally, with the highest rates occurring in sub-Saharan Africa (49). When the mother passes the infection to her child during pregnancy, childbirth, or breast-feeding, this is termed vertical transmission. The risk increases if the virus load is high, HIV disease is advanced, and the CD4 cell count is low in the mother (50). Much evidence suggests that mother-to-child transmission occurs at least 50% of the time near or during delivery (49).

To reduce the risk of perinatal transmission of HIV, zidovudine, commonly known as AZT, has been given to HIV-positive women from the 14th week of pregnancy until delivery and then to the neonate for 6 weeks (50). Following this protocol, Connor et al (51) showed that zidovudine reduced perinatal transmission by approximately 70% in a study of the AIDS Clinical Trials Group.

Researchers have not confirmed that HIV infection is inevitable in infants breast-fed by seropositive women. Nonetheless, the virus has been detected in breast milk. Studies of the link between breast-feeding and the risk of vertical transmission of HIV-1 have reported conflicting results (52).

In countries where malnutrition and infectious diseases are primary causes of infant mortality, the World Health Organization (WHO) and the United Nations (UN) recommend breast-feeding because infants face a greater risk of dying of other causes than from HIV infection contracted through breast milk (52). However, in developed countries where the standards of sanitation are high and the water supply is safe, the WHO and the UN advise HIV-infected women not to breast-feed. The American Academy of Pediatrics supports this position as well.

Decisions about whether to breast-feed should be based on an evaluation of factors affecting HIV transmission and priorities for neonatal health and survival (52). An informed decision depends on the benefits and risks of breast-feeding vs bottle feeding and the clinical and laboratory status of the mother and child. Human milk banks may be an option to reduce transmission risk (Figure 3-3). In developed countries the decision to breast-feed should rest with the mother and her physician.

## Summary

Managing the dietary problems that each HIV-infected patient faces is a challenge for the health care professional, caregiver, and patient. Nutrition problems that affect appetite and weight require the dietitian to educate patients about the need for healthy eating, including appropriate food choices, vitamin and mineral supplementation, and adherence to food safety guidelines. Guidelines for managing HIV symptoms of dietary relevance such as anorexia, nausea and vomiting, mouth pain and swallowing difficulties, taste alterations, and diarrhea may require a special focus. Oral nutritional supplements are sometimes necessary, and complementary therapies may represent viable treatment options. Client-centered nutrition counseling will help to ensure a cooperative working relationship between the client and caregiver. Finally, the nutri-

**FIGURE 3-3 Breast-feeding Decision Tree: A decision tree to help clinicians evaluate risks and benefits of breast-feeding in HIV-infected women in developed countries**

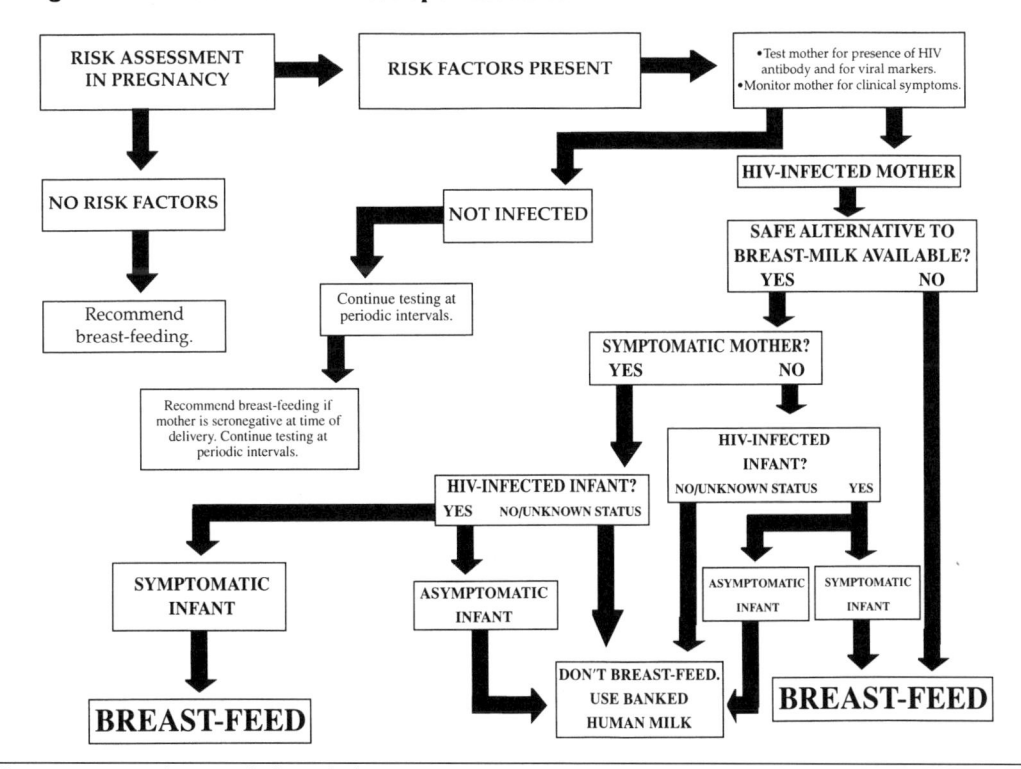

Source: Black RF. Transmission of HIV-1 in the breast-feeding process. *J Am Diet Assoc.* 1996;96:267-274. Used with permission.

tion needs of HIV-infected women may require all of the above expertise in addition to special considerations for the requirements of pregnancy and lactation.

## References

1. Coodley GO, Nelson HD, Loveless MO, Folk C. Beta-carotene in HIV infection. *J Acquired Immune Defic Syndromes.* 1993;6:272-276.
2. Kotler DP, Tierney AR, Wang J, Pierson RN: Magnitude of body cell mass depletion and the timing of death from wasting in AIDS. *Am J Clin Nutr.* 1989;50:444-447.
3. The Chicago Dietetic Association and The South Suburban Dietetic Association: *Manual of Clinical Dietetics.* 5th ed. Chicago, Ill: American Dietetic Association; 1996.
4. Hellerstein MK. Pathophysiology of lean body mass wasting and nutrient unresponsiveness in HIV/AIDS: therapeutic implications. In: *Proceedings of 1992 International Conference on Nutrition and HIV/AIDS.* Chicago, Ill: PAAC; 1993:17-25.
5. HIV/AIDS Medical Nutrition Therapy Protocol. *Medical Nutrition Therapy Across the Continuum of Care.* Chicago, Ill: The American Dietetic Association; 1996.
6. Position of The American Dietetic Association and The Canadian Dietetic Association: Nutrition intervention in the care of persons with human immunodeficiency virus infection. *J Am Diet Assoc.* 1994;94:1042-1045.
7. Flaskerud JH: AIDS and traditional food therapies. In: Watson RR, ed: *Nutrition and AIDS.* Ann Arbor, Mich: CRC Press; 1994:235-247.
8. *Dietetics Online.* (http://www.dietetics.com).
9. Salomon SB, Davis M, Fields-Gardner C: *Living Well with HIV and AIDS: A Guide to Healthy Eating.* Chicago, Ill: American Dietetic Association; 1993.
10. *Health Care and HIV: Nutritional Guide for Providers and Clients.* Vienna, Va: Bureau of Primary Health Care, US Department of Health and Human Services; 1996.
11. Coodley GO, Loveless MO, Nelson HD, Coodley MK. Endocrine function in the wasting syndrome. *J AIDS.* 1994;7:46-51.
12. Miller ARO, Griffin GE, Batman P, Farquar C, Forster SM, Pinching AJ, Harris JRW. Jejunal mucosal architecture and fat absorption in male homosexuals with human immunodeficiency virus. *Qu J Med.* 1988;260:1009-1091.
13. Thomson C. Specialized nutrition support. In: Watson RR, ed: *Nutrition and AIDS.* Ann Arbor, Mich: CRC Press; 1994:201-213.
14. Van Roenn JH, Armstrong D, Kotler DP, Cohn DL, Klimas NG, Tchekmedyian NS, Cone L, Brennan PJ, Weitzman SA. Megestrol acetate in patients with AIDS-related cachexia. *Ann Intern Med.* 1994;121:393-399.
15. Graham KK, Mikolich, Fisher AE, Posner MR, Dudley MN. Pharmacologic evaluation of megestrol acetate oral suspension in cachectic AIDS patients. *J Acquired Immune Defic Syndromes.* 1994;7:580-586.
16. Brady MT, Koranyi KI, Hunkler JA. Megestrol acetate for treatment of anorexia associated with human immunodeficiency virus infection in children. *Pediatr Infect Dis J.* 1994;13:754-756.
17. Novak J, Barkin JS. Megace for AIDS cachexia: food for thought. *Am J Gastroenterol.* 1995;90:1180-1181.
18. Hengge UR, Brockmeyer NH: Megestrol for AIDS-related anorexia. *Ann Intern Med.* 1995;122:879. Letter.
19. Tchekmedyian NS. Clinical approaches to nutritional support in cancer. *Curr Opin Oncol.* 1993;5:633-638.
20. Mauer M: Megestrol for AIDS-related anorexia. *Ann Intern Med.* 1995;122:880. Letter.
21. Nerad JL, Gorbach SL. Nutritional aspects of HIV infection: management of infection in HIV disease. *Infect Dis Clin North Am.* 1994;8:499-515.
22. Conant M, Roy D, Shepard KV, Plasse TF. Dronabinol enhances appetite and

controls weight loss in HIV patients. In: *Programs and Abstracts of the Proceedings of the American Society of Clinical Oncology.* Houston, Tex: American Society of Clinical Oncology; 1991.
23. Plasse TF, Gorter RW, Krasnow SH, Lane M, Shepard KV. Recent clinical experience with dronabinol. *Pharmacol Biochem Behav.* 1991;40:695-700.
24. Beal JE, Olson R, Laubenstein L, Morales JO, Bellman P, Yangco B, Lefkowitz L, Plasse TF, Shepard KV. Dronabinol as a treatment for anorexia associated with weight loss in patients with AIDS. *J Pain Symptom Manage.* 1995;10:89-92.
25. Cook PP. Megestrol for AIDS-related anorexia. *Ann Intern Med.* 1995;122:879-880. Letter.
26. Bahl S. Drug-induced nutritional complications and their management. In: Bahl S, Hickson JF Jr. *Nutritional Care for HIV-Positive Persons: A Manual for Individuals and Their Caregivers.* Ann Arbor, Mich: CRC Press; 1995.
27. Abrams B, Duncan D, Hertz-Picciotto IH: A prospective study of dietary intake and acquired immune deficiency syndrome in HIV-seropositive homosexual men. *J AIDS.* 1993;6:949-958.
28. Tang AM, Graham NMH, Kirby AJ, McCall LC, Willett WC, Saah AJ. Dietary micronutrient intake and risk of progression to human immunodeficiency virus type 1 (HIV-1)-infected homosexual men. *Am J Epidemiol.* 1993;138:937-951.
29. Tang AM, Graham NMH, Semba RD, Saah AJ. Association between serum vitamin A and E levels and HIV-1 disease progression. *AIDS.* 1997;11:613-620.
30. Wang H, Cao G, Prior RL. Total antioxidant capacity of fruits. *J Agric Food Chem.* 1996;44:701-705.
31. Cao G, Sofic E, Prior RL. Antioxidant capacity of tea and common vegetables. *J Agric Food Chem.* 1996;44:3426-3431.
32. Bell SJ, Forse RA, *Positive Nutrition for HIV infection & AIDS.* Minneapolis, Miin: Chronimed Publishing; 1996.
33. Lehmann RH. *Cooking for Life.* New York, NY: Dell Publishing; 1997.
34. Brodsky M. Paying lip service to calories: oral nutrition supplements. *Positively Aware.* March 1993:22.
35. Barrett S. Immunoquackery. In: Barrett S, Jarvis WT, eds. *The Health Robbers: A Close Look at Quackery in America.* Buffalo, NY: Prometheus Books; 1993:155-157.
36. Vaghefi SB, Castellon-Vogel EA. Nutrition and AIDS: an introductory chapter. In: Watson RR, ed: *Nutrition and AIDS.* Ann Arbor, Mich: CRC Press; 1994:1-16.
37. Herbert V. Vitamin pushers and food quacks. In: Barrett S, Jarvis WT, eds. *The Health Robbers: A Close Look at Quackery in America.* Buffalo, NY: Prometheus Books; 1993:28.
38. Tyler VE. *The Honest Herbal.* 3rd ed. Binghamton, NY: Haworth Press; 1993.
39. Dwyer JT, Bye RL, Holt PL, Lauze SR. Unproven nutrition therapies for AIDS: what is the evidence? *Nutr Today.* March/April 1988:25-33.
40. Zwicky JF, Hafner AW, Barrett S, Jarvis WT. *Reader's Guide to Alternative Health Methods.* Chicago, Ill: American Medical Association; 1993:9-10.
41. Licavoli L, Hahn NI. Dietetics goes into therapy. *J Am Diet Assoc.* 1995; 95:751-752.
42. Abdale F. *Community-Based Nutrition Support for People Living With HIV and AIDS. A Technical Assistance Manual.* New York, NY: God's Love We Deliver; 1995.
43. Snetselaar LG. *Nutrition Counseling Skills for Medical Nutrition Therapy.* Gaithersburg, Md: Aspen Publishers; 1997.
44. Bahl S. HIV-infection in women, infants, and children. In: Bahl S, Hickson JF Jr. *Nutritional Care for HIV-Positive Persons: A Manual for Individuals and Their Caregivers.* Ann Arbor, Mich: CRC Press; 1995: chapter 8.
45. Henderson C. AIDS slowing but not among women and blacks. *AIDS Weekly Plus.* Nov 11, 1996:10.
46. Centers for Disease Control and Prevention. *HIV/AIDS Surveillance Rep.* 1996;8. Midyear edition reported through June 1996 (available also by Internet: http://www.cdc.gov).
47. UNAIDS and WHO. *The Global Epidemic,* December 1996. Based on *The Status and Trends of the Global HIV/AIDS Pandemic,* Vancouver, Canada, July 5-6, 1996 (http://www.who.gov).

48. Subcommittee on Nutritional Status and Weight Gain During Pregnancy, Subcommittee on Dietary Intake and Nutrient Supplements During Pregnancy, Committee on Nutritional Status During Pregnancy and Lactation, Food and Nutrition Board, Institute of Medicine, National Academy of Sciences. *Nutrition During Pregnancy: Part I, Weight Gain, Part II, Nutrient Supplements.* Washington, DC: National Academy Press; 1990.
49. Bulterys M, Goedert JJ. From biology to sexual behavior—towards the prevention of mother-to-child transmission of HIV. *AIDS.* 1996;10:1287-1289. Editorial.
50. Bryson YJ. Perinatal HIV-1 transmission: recent advances and therapeutic interventions. *AIDS.* 1996;10(suppl 3):S33-S42.
51. Connor EM, Sperling RS, Gelber R, Kiselev P, Scott G, O'Sullivan MJ, Van Dyke R, Bey M, Shearer W, Jacobson RL. Reduction of maternal-infant transmission of human immunodeficiency virus type 1 with zidovudine treatment. *N Engl J Med.* 1994;31:1173-1180.
52. Black RF. Transmission of HIV-1 in the breast-feeding process. *J Am Diet Assoc.* 1996;96:267-274.

# 4
# Enteral and Parenteral Nutrition Strategies

The compromised nutritional status of people with the acquired immunodeficiency syndrome (AIDS) or other disease states caused by the human immunodeficiency virus (HIV) is demonstrated by problems such as rapid and unintentional weight loss, malabsorption syndrome, recurrent infective processes, and multiple nutritional deficiencies. In an effort to control malnutrition associated with these problems, specialized options for nutrition support must be instituted when oral intake fails or is at risk of failure to produce the desired outcomes. Weight gain, improved visceral and somatic protein stores, and an improved ability to perform activities of daily living are representative of these outcomes.

Advances in enteral and parenteral nutrition over the past 25 years have allowed clinicians to broaden their scope of practice to include nutrition support for patients with HIV disease. The purpose of this chapter is to briefly review the current literature in the area of specialized nutrition support of HIV-positive patients and to provide the appropriate information and tools needed to initiate, monitor, and evaluate nutrition support. Initially, goals for nutrition support will be reviewed, including fluid, energy, protein, and micronutrient requirements. Next, selected topics for managing and monitoring enteral and parenteral nutrition support will be discussed. The final topic addressed will be the role of the dietitian on the nutrition support team.

## Goals for Nutrition Support

Goals and methods may be similar to those for other patients requiring nutrition support, but additional considerations may come into play for patients with HIV disease. Since HIV disease is characterized as a chronic inflammatory disease, many alterations in the metabolism of nutrients may indicate the need for conservative and stepwise management. This approach may help prevent the detrimental effects of overfeeding and other metabolic compromises to an already stressed patient.

The following goals (summarized in Table 4-1) may be met by nutrition support in conjunction with other therapies: minimize catabolism, replenish lost nutrients and body cell mass (BCM), improve host resistance, improve pharmacologic response, preserve gut function, and maintain or improve psychosocial well-being. It is preferable that patients be assessed individually using their own baseline data as usual values and starting points. A tailored nutrition care plan is then formulated to achieve these goals with consideration of other medical strategies. Enteral and parenteral feeding may be a necessary component in the achievement of these goals as either a primary or adjunctive nutrition therapy.

Two types of malnutrition are observed in HIV-infected patients: starvation-related and cachexia-related wasting (1, 2). Resulting from voluntary or involuntary reduced food intake, the starvation-type wasting occurs in clinically stable patients without an opportunistic infection. These patients have a good response to nutrition support. Accurate assessment of gastrointestinal function and lean body mass is important in treatment of starvation-related wasting syndrome. However, patients with cachexia-related wasting have a poor response even when their energy requirements are exceeded unless the underlying opportunistic infection is treated (1).

A paucity of research exists in the area of specialized nutrition support in HIV disease and a common complaint is that study populations tend to be small. Generally, patients demonstrate an ability to regain weight but not always at a clinically significant rate. Studies of patients with systemic illnesses suggest a more significant increase in body fat rather than a more desirable increase in protein stores. The subgroup of patients who do not replenish protein stores through nutrition support may be categorized as "nonresponders" (1-3). Five outcomes are generally accepted as indicative of the effectiveness of nutrition support: repletion of BCM, improvement in physiologic function, reduced length of hospitalization, improved quality of life, and prolonged survival (Table 4-2).

### TABLE 4-1  Goals of Nutrition Support in HIV Disease

**Goal**

Minimize loss of protein stores with adequate protein support

Replenish lost nutrients during postcatabolic phase rehabilitation

Improve host response with adequate fluids, energy, and protein

Improve pharmacologic response through nutritional rehabilitation and maintenance

Preserve gut function through fluid and nutrient stimulation and maintenance of gastrointestinal lining and function

Maintain and improve psychosocial well-being

**TABLE 4-2 Outcomes for Nutrition Support Effectiveness**

| Outcome | Monitors |
|---|---|
| Repletion of body cell mass | Weight, body mass index, anthropometry, bio-electrical impedance analysis, other tests or estimates of body cell mass |
| Improved physiologic function | Strength or endurance tests, improved tolerance and response to medications, specific functional tests, hydration |
| Reduced length of hospital stay | Actual length of stay compared with average length of stay |
| Improved quality of life | Quality of life measurements or tools, independent living with improved ability in activities of daily living and/or instrumental activities of daily living |
| Prolonged survival | Actual survival compared with average survival with matched clinical profile |

## Nutrition Assessment

The first step in nutrition support is to conduct a thorough nutrition assessment. Assessment includes anthropometric and biochemical evaluations, a complete review of medical and dietary histories, and a nutrition-oriented physical examination (to determine the presence of nutrition-related signs and symptoms of deficiency or excess). A review of the medical record should focus on past medical history, medication use, biochemical trends, previous dietary restrictions, findings of previous nutrient intake analyses, and a complete diagnostic history. For a more in-depth review of the specifics of assessment, see Chapter 2.

## Individualized Nutrition Support

Dietitians use nutrition assessment data to estimate individual needs. Emphasis typically is placed on fluid, energy, and protein requirements, since these patients may exhibit dehydration and protein-energy malnutrition. Ongoing monitors of the efficacy of therapy should specifically address desired outcomes and should minimize complications and undesirable side effects.

### FLUID REQUIREMENTS

It is essential to determine and monitor fluid requirements in conjunction with the provision of nutrition support. To calculate fluid needs, 30 to 35 mL/kg of dry body weight per day, plus allowances of insensible and other losses, will give a reasonable assessment of fluid needs. Factors that add to insensible losses and increase fluid requirements include diarrhea, fistulas, fever, open wounds, artificial ventilation, dry climate, exercise, increased respiration, and copious night sweats.

The dietitian should consider free water levels in enteral and parenteral feedings when developing a nutrition support regimen. For nutrition support purposes, daily estimates are generally 1 mL/kcal.

More concentrated formulations may be used when volume poses a problem. Provided that the patient's fluid status permits, addition of sterile water is recommended when the tube feeding or parenteral solution does not provide adequate free water.

Since feedings can override thirst mechanisms, it will be important to monitor for overhydration and dehydration as well as weight changes. The consequences of fluid overload include hypervolemia and congestive heart failure. Consider the use of diuretics, presence of renal insufficiency, and accuracy of data collection methods when evaluating fluid input and output measurements. Symptoms to monitor include dyspnea and tachycardia. Daily weights and vital signs can be clues to dehydration and overhydration. Laboratory data to monitor include serum sodium, serum (blood) urea nitrogen (BUN), potassium, phosphorus, calcium, glucose, chloride, albumin, selenium, zinc, magnesium, carbon dioxide, creatinine, alkaline phosphatase, lipase, amylase, bilirubin, and total protein. Whenever possible, correction of abnormal values should be accomplished by addressing the underlying problem. Adding or subtracting the substrate under question in the enteral or parenteral form may be necessary to correct abnormal laboratory data related to hydration (Table 4-3).

## ENERGY REQUIREMENTS

As with other acutely or critically ill patients, the energy requirements for patients with HIV disease to achieve anabolism generally fall in the range of 30 to 40 kcal/kg of actual body weight per day, dependent on the presence of an opportunistic infection. If a patient is more than 20% over ideal body weight (IBW), adjusted weight should be calculated as follows: (Actual Weight - IBW) x 0.25 + IBW. Actual body weight is used if the patient is at dry weight and below IBW. The Harris-Benedict equation may also be used with appropriate injury and activity factors. It is essential to use good clinical judgment on the timing and advancement of support as well as the transitions between feeding methods to provide metabolic stabilization and maintenance to nutritional rehabilitation.

As with other disease states, the clinician should carefully monitor for overfeeding to avoid additional complications and organ function compromise. These monitors can include weight, acid-base balance measures, electrolyte balance, and organ function (renal, hepatic, and pulmonary).

In the presence of fever and infection, energy expenditure is clearly increased and energy provision should be adjusted accordingly. However, in severely wasted patients the initial goal is metabolic support and stabilization. It may be judicious to start with a minimum kilocalorie level of 15-20 kcal/kg of actual body weight and progress to a goal maintenance or rehabilitation level in a stepwise fashion. Bioelectrical impedance analysis or other sensitive estimation of BCM is helpful to determine the amount of tissue that requires energy support. Each step or advance in nutrition support should be monitored closely for complications and for signs associated with overfeeding. These include hypertriglyceridemia, increased liver function tests, hypercapnia, and hyperglycemia.

### TABLE 4-3 Biochemical Alterations Associated With Enteral and Parenteral Nutrition Support[a]

| Key Monitor | Monitoring Frequency | Cause | Nutrition Prescription |
|---|---|---|---|
| **Serum Urea Nitrogen (BUN)** | | | |
| Decreased | qd 5-7 d, then 3 times weekly | Malnutrition | Provide nutrition support especially with protein |
| | | Fluid overload | Restrict fluids |
| Increased (azotemia) | | Dehydration, renal failure, excess protein administration | Increase fluids, restrict protein based on creatinine clearance and use or disuse of dialysis |
| **Creatinine** | | | |
| Decreased | qd 5-7 d, then 3 times weekly | Malnutrition, fluid overload | Reassess nitrogen (N) balance |
| Increased | | Dehydration, renal failure | Reassess N balance |
| **Serum Bicarbonate** | | | |
| Decreased (acidosis) | qd 5-7 d, then 3 times weekly | Metabolic acidosis: diarrhea, sepsis, renal failure, respiratory alkalosis | Medically correct underlying problem, provide Na+/K+ in acetate form 1 mEq/kg per day |
| | | | Provide Na+/K+ in acetate form 1 mEq/kg per day |
| Increased (alkalosis) | | Metabolic alkalosis: nasogastric suction | Antacids |
| **Zinc** | | | |
| Decreased (hypozincemia) | If available, check when ↑ losses are suspected and after treatment | Diarrhea, small-bowel fistulas, AIDS, burns, diuretics | Zinc (Zn) supplement as $ZnSO_4$ approximately 12 mg/L of diarrhea |
| **Liver Function Tests** | | | |
| Increased | Weekly | Fatty liver infiltration, cholestasis, ↑ glycogen deposition, essential fatty acid deficiency | Minimize dextrose load <5 mg/kg per minute, use gastrointestinal tract or cycle TPN, provide exogenous lipids, supplement with small amount of corn oil via gastrointestinal tract |
| | | Choline deficiency | Choline supplementation |
| **Potassium (K)** | | | |
| Decreased (hypokalemia) | qd 5-7 d, then weekly | Inadequate K+ intake, diuretics, diarrhea | Provide K+ supplement |
| Increased (hyperkalemia) | qd 5-7 d, then 3 times weekly | Renal failure, excess replacement therapy, resolution of problem associated with deficiency (ie, no diarrhea after refeeding response), metabolic acidosis secondary to renal insufficiency, insulin deficiency | Restrict K+, monitor K+ runs and supplements, provide insulin |

TABLE 4-3  Biochemical Alterations Associated With Enteral and Parenteral Nutrition Support[a] (Continued)

| Key Monitor | Monitoring Frequency | Cause | Nutrition Prescription |
|---|---|---|---|
| **Sodium (Na)** | | | |
| Decreased (hyponatremia) | qd 5-7 d, then 3 times weekly | Fluid overload, deficiency (gastrointestinal losses), long-term TF with low Na+ product | Restrict fluids, check urine Na+, add NaCl to formula or change to higher Na+ formula, restrict fluids, consult pharmacist |
| | | SIADH, diuretics | |
| Increased (hypernatremia) | | Dehydration, excess administration (TPN, TF, IVF), free water loss secondary to drug interaction | Increase fluid load, restrict Na+, ↑ fluids |
| **Phosphorus** | | | |
| Decreased (hypophosphatemia) | qd 3 d, then 1-2 times weekly | Refeeding syndrome | Replace as Na+ or K+ phosphate, either IV or by mouth |
| | | Dextrose, CHO administration, excess phosphate binders, large-dose insulin therapy | ↓ CHO load and replace kilocalories as fat, discontinue or ↓ phosphate binders, phosphorus supplementation |
| Increased (hyperphosphatemia) | | Renal failure, excess replacement therapy | Reduce or discontinue phosphorus in TPN or TF, use phosphorus binders, discontinue phosphorous replacement |
| **Magnesium (Mg)** | | | |
| Decreased (hypomagnesemia) | qd 3 d, then 1-2 times weekly | Refeeding | Supplement IV or via TF as $MgSO_4$ or $MgO_2$ |
| | | Medications (amphotericin, cyclosporine, diuretics) | Mg++ supplement |
| | | diarrhea | Replace estimated losses |
| Increased (hypermagnesemia) | | Renal failure, excess replacement therapy, Mg++ containing antacids | Restrict or change TF or TPN formula |
| | | | Discontinue or ↓ replacement, monitor medicine, consult pharmacist |
| **Calcium (Ca)** | | | |
| Decreased (hypocalcemia) | 2 times weekly, then once weekly | Pancreatitis, low serum albumin, inadequate Mg++, inadequate Ca++ (especially during phosphorous supplementation or vitamin D deficiency) | Treat medically, calculate correct Ca++, ↑ Mg++, ↑ Ca++ or ↓ phosphorous, evaluate adequate intake of vitamin D |
| Increased (hypercalcemia) | | Metabolic bone disease, excess Ca++ and/or vitamin D | Medical therapy: diuresis, delete vitamin D and/or ↑ phosphorus, ↓ or delete Ca from solution |

## TABLE 4-3 Biochemical Alterations Associated With Enteral and Parenteral Nutrition Support[a] (Continued)

| Key Monitor | Monitoring Frequency | Cause | Nutrition Prescription |
|---|---|---|---|
| **Nitrogen Balance** | Every 7-10 d | | |
| Positive | | Adequate provision of protein | Provide protein based on calculations |
| Negative | | Inadequate provision of kilocalories or protein | ↑ Protein, kilocalories, adjust kilocalorie-to-nitrogen ratio |
| Inaccurate | | Renal failure, improper or inaccurate collection, <8 hour collection | Use urea kinetics, provide in-service, note that literature variable |
| **Weight** | | | |
| Increased | qd | Anabolism | Decrease kilocalories |
| Decreased | | Catabolism | Increase kilocalories |
| Fluctuates | | Fluid shifts | Adjust fluid volume |
| **Albumin** | | | |
| Decreased (hypoalbuminemia) | Weekly | Catabolism, liver failure, surgery, acute stress, fluid overload | ↑ Protein, obtain UUN, ↓ protein with encephalopathy, ↑ protein |
| | | | Decrease fluids, diuresis |
| Increased (hyperalbuminemia) | | Dehydration, renal failure | ↑ Fluids, adjust protein load based on clinical status (urinary output, dialysis, creatinine clearance, UUN) |
| **Prealbumin** | | | |
| Decreased | 2 times weekly | Catabolism | ↑ Protein, adjust kilocalorie-to-nitrogen ratio |
| Increased | | Renal failure | Adjust protein load based on clinical status |
| **Triglycerides** | | | |
| Decreased (hypotriglyceridemia) | qd 3 d, then 2 times weekly | Malnutrition | No treatment to feed, lipid ≤2.5 g/kg |
| Increased (hypertriglyceremia) | | End-stage AIDS, CAD, diabetes mellitus, fat mobilization | ↓ Saturated fat, ↓ total fat, provide adequate nutrition support |
| | | Carnitine deficiency | Provide carnitine |
| **Glucose** | | | |
| Decreased (hypoglycemia) | At least qd 5 d, then 3 times weekly | Excess insulin, "rebound" hypoglycemia, abrupt discontinuation of TPN | ↓ Insulin load, avoid long-acting insulin, wean gradually |
| Increased (hyperglycemia) | | Stress response, infection treated medically, medications, diabetes mellitus, cancer, excess dextrose infusion | Adjust insulin, ↓ CHO kilocalories, ↓ total kilocalories, check dextrose infusion = 5-7 mg/kg per minute, ↑ free water |

[a]qd indicates every day; {(↑)}, increase or increased; {(↓)}, decrease or decreased; TF, tube feeding; SIADH, syndrome of inadequate diuretic hormone; TPN, total parenteral nutrition; IVF, intravenous fluids; CHO, carbohydrates; IV, intravenous; UUN, urine urea nitrogen; CAD, coronary artery disease.

Patients infected with HIV who have a prolonged reduction in energy intake or decreased absorption of nutrients may experience a reduction in metabolic rate. In the absence of systemic illness, these patients may achieve a positive energy balance with a relative reduction in estimated energy requirements. In other cases, a positive energy balance may require administration of up to 45 to 60 kcal/kg to overcome compromised nutrition. Energy requirements must be adjusted on an individual basis based on changes in clinical status and on clinical response to nutrition therapy.

Routine calorie counts, laboratory value evaluation, and weight monitoring will help to assess trends and reassess needs. Metabolic cart equipment may provide a more accurate method to estimate energy requirements during nutrition support or any acute medical events (see Appendix B); however, this equipment may not yet be readily available for use by many nutrition professionals.

## PROTEIN REQUIREMENTS

Protein requirements and tolerance may vary significantly depending on acute events and organ function. Hospitalized HIV-positive patients receiving specialized nutrition support may require 1 to 2.5 g of protein per kilogram of actual body weight per day. During acute phases, metabolic stabilization will include a goal of positive nitrogen balance to contribute to the amino acid pool, in the hope of blunting severe catabolic response to stress.

Special attention should be given to renal and hepatic function, and appropriate reductions in protein load estimations should be made as indicated. The clinician should closely monitor for protein tolerance and signs of anabolism, so that strategy adjustments may be made in a timely manner.

Laboratory indicators of protein adequacy should be interpreted with caution. Albumin has been the standard measure used for the evaluation of visceral protein status. However, albumin alone has limitations as a nutritional status indicator due to a fairly long half-life (18 to 21 days), and the fluid shifts to extravascular space during acute phases of infection. Prealbumin has a shorter half-life (2.5 to 3 days) but also is affected by an acute phase response of the liver during infection. During the acute phase of the inflammatory process, a repolarization of protein synthesis occurs. Levels of albumin, transferrin, and other transport proteins decrease, whereas levels of C-reactive protein, alpha-1-acid glycoprotein, ceruloplasmin, and fibrinogen increase. These fluid shifts have a dilutional effect on visceral protein indexes. Transferrin, however, may be falsely elevated in the presence of low serum iron stores, a common characteristic seen in HIV. A urine urea nitrogen measure used in a nitrogen balance study may be valuable to further assess protein needs. An optimal nitrogen balance in stress might be from 0 to +2 g, whereas the patient whose goal is rehabilitation may benefit from achieving positive nitrogen balance by an extra 3 to 5 g of nitrogen or 20 to 30 g more of protein daily.

## MICRONUTRIENTS

Patients with HIV infection have an increased frequency of metabolic alterations. These changes may result in apparent deficient levels of micronutrients, especially in the face of acute illness or increased stress. Of patients tested in a longitudinal prospective cohort study, laboratory indexes of micronutrients were significantly below normal ranges in advanced HIV disease and were associated with wasting syndrome (4, 5). Since many micronutrient laboratory values may be altered in metabolic dysfunction, caution should be taken in the interpretation of these laboratory values in planning for specialized nutrition support. Close monitoring for detrimental side effects is as crucial in administration of nutrients as it is for drug regimens. Although many tests for vitamin and mineral levels may not be readily available for assessment, the diet history, clinical examination, and medical status evaluation should help the clinician to determine the need for supplementation.

It remains to be seen whether the US Recommended Dietary Allowances (RDA) level of nutrient provision will be adequate to correct existing deficiencies or maintain adequate levels in the HIV population, especially in the presence of opportunistic infection or disease progression. It is also unclear whether normal ranges are even appropriate in HIV. Studies on nutrient deficiency and supplementation suggest that additional supplementation with zinc; selenium; vitamins C, B-12, and B-6; or folate may be indicated above the usual dietary intake (6-8). It is costly and difficult, however, to accurately assess micronutrient deficiencies in individual patients. Supplementation of micronutrients is a reasonable practice within safe limits if closely monitored. For example, zinc may be provided in the oral form as 25 mg or less of zinc sulfate or in the parenteral form as 2.5 to 4 mg of elemental zinc. A recommended selenium dosage would be 0.87 $\mu$g/kg weight.

## Enteral Feeding

The type of feeding selected depends on gastrointestinal function and access as well as the patient and the health care team's assessment, preferences, and formulary. Figure 4-1 shows a clinical decision tree that may be used in the decision-making process. Table 4-4 lists diagnoses that may justify the use of nutrition support. Indications for various feeding routes are presented in Table 4-5.

### FORMULA SELECTION AND CHARACTERISTICS

Currently more than 100 commercial adult oral/enteral formulas are available. Each is specifically indicated for routes of administration and nutritional properties. The enteral formulas fall into two major classifications based on their protein content: standard and special. The standard formulas consist of intact protein, such as pureed meat, egg albumin, and soy lactalbumin, and are intended for patients with normal gut function (9). The special enteral formulas are hydrolyzed, containing protein as amino acids or polypeptides, or they have alternate sources of fats or are higher or lower in certain nutrients to provide a desired effect.

**FIGURE 4-1  Decision Tree for Nutrition Support in HIV Disease and AIDS**

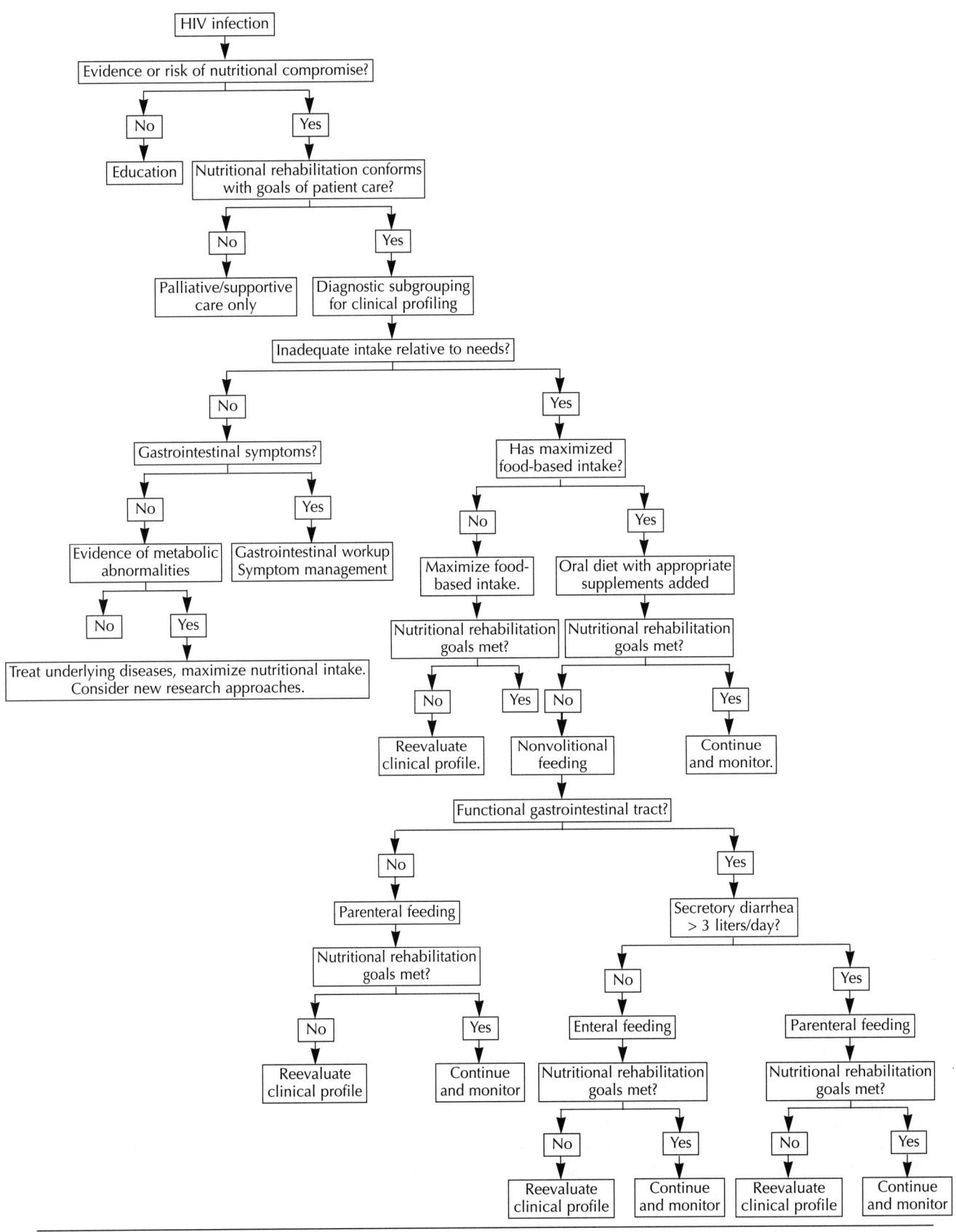

**TABLE 4-4  HIV-Related Medical Conditions That Justify Nutrition Support**

**Enteral Feedings**
AIDS enteropathy
Anorexia—failure of volitional oral intake
Coma
Dysphagia (severe)
Idiopathic weight loss
Intubation or respirator ventilation
Mental status changes resulting in inadequate intake and malnutrition
Achlorhydria (severe)
Chronic pancreatitis

**Parenteral Feedings**
AIDS enteropathy
Cryptosporidiosis with persistent diarrhea
Cytomegalovirus with persistent secretory diarrhea
Herpes simplex virus with extensive lesions in perianal area
Intractable emesis
Distal obstructions of gastrointestinal tract from neoplasms and Kaposi's sarcoma
*Mycobacterium avium-intracellulare* with persistent diarrhea
Acute pancreatitis
Severe protein-energy malnutrition

These formulas are used for patients with compromised gut function or other special needs. Table 4-6 shows a sampling of each category of enteral formulas and the volume required to meet the RDA for micronutrients. Modular formulas, which vary according to the composition of individual nutrients, are reviewed in Table 4-7.

The key factors to consider in the formula selection process include the following: gut function, formula availability, patient acceptance and tolerance, nutritional requirements, feeding route (gastric vs small bowel), administration technique (bolus vs gravity and continuous vs cyclic), duration of support, and cost. No one enteral product is appropriate for use in all patients with HIV disease. With many patients, the

**TABLE 4-5  Enteral Feeding Routes and Indications**

| Route | Indications |
| --- | --- |
| Nasogastric | Appropriate for short-term, alert, ambulatory HIV-positive patients at low risk for aspiration and in patients in whom bolus feeding is preferable (ie, patients being considered for short-term nutrition support at home) |
| Nasoduodenal | Appropriate for short-term feeding in HIV-positive patients with increased risk of aspiration (ie, altered mental status, neurologic impairment) and in whom continuous administration of formula is preferable (ie, intolerant to bolus feeding, nonambulatory) |
| Percutaneous endoscopic gastrostomy (PEG) | Same indications as for nasogastric tube; also necessary when oral or esophageal lesions preclude the nasal route |
| Percutaneous endoscopic jejunostosmy (PEJ) | Same indications as for nasoduodenal; needle catheter jejunostomy tube should be used only with defined or elemental formulas to avoid clogging |

### TABLE 4-6  Sampling of Enteral Products

| Indication | Formula/Manufacturer[a] | Kilocalories/Volume (mL) to Meet 100% RDA[b] for Micronutrients |
|---|---|---|
| Standard | Attain/Sherwood Medical | 1,250/1,250 |
|  | Compleat Modified/Novartis | 1,402/1,500 |
|  | Ensure/Ross | 1,780/1,887 |
|  | Isocal/Mead Johnson | 1,783/1,890 |
|  | Osmolite/Ross | 1,780/1,887 |
|  | Sustacal/Mead Johnson | 1,783/1,890 |
| Critical illness/ stress | Advera/Ross | 1,939/1,515 |
|  | Crucial/Nestle | 1,500/1,000 |
|  | ImmunAid/McGaw | 2,000/2,000 |
|  | Impact/Novartis | 1,500/1,500 |
|  | Isosource VHN/Novartis | 1,250/1,250 |
|  | L-Emental Plus/Nutrition Medical | 1,800/1,800 |
|  | Peptamen HP/Nestle | 1,500/1,500 |
|  | Perative/Ross | 888/1,155 |
|  | Promote/Ross | 1,000/1,000 |
|  | Pro-Peptide VHN/Nutrition Medical | 1,500/1,500 |
|  | Protain XL/Sherwood Medical | 1,250/1,250 |
|  | Reabilan HN/Nestle | 1,995/1,500 |
|  | Replete/Nestle | 1,000/1,000 |
|  | Traumacal/Mead Johnson | 3,000/2,000 |
|  | Vivonex Plus/Novartis | 1,800/1,800 |
| Impaired fat absorption | AlitraQ/Ross | 1,500/1,500 |
|  | Criticare HN/Mead Johnson | 1,783/1,890 |
|  | ImmunAid/McGaw | 2,000/2,000 |
|  | L-Emental/Nutrition Medical | 2,000/2,000 |
|  | Lipisorb/Mead Johnson | 1,481/2,000 |
|  | Peptamen/Nestle | 1,500/1,500 |
|  | Pro-Peptide VHN/Nutrition Medical | 1,500/1,500 |
|  | Reabilan/Nestle | 2,000/2,000 |
|  | SandoSource Peptide/Novartis | 1,750/1,750 |
|  | Vital HN/Ross | 1,500/1,500 |
|  | Vivonex TEN/Novartis | 2,000/2,000 |
| Volume/ fluid restriction | Comply/Sherwood Medical | 667/1,000 |
|  | Deliver 2/Mead Johnson | 667/1,000 |
|  | Magnacal/Sherwood Medical | 667/1,000 |
|  | TwoCal HN/Ross | 475/950 |
| Renal insufficiency | Amin-Aid/McGaw | Does not meet RDA for vitamins/minerals |
|  | Nepro/Ross | 474/947 |
|  | Suplena/Ross | 474/947 |
| Hepatic insufficiency | HepaticAid II/McGaw | Does not meet RDA for vitamins/minerals |
|  | Magnacal/Sherwood Medical | 500/1,000 |
|  | NutriHep/Nestle | 1,500/1,000 |
|  | L-Emental Hepatic/Nutrition Medical | Does not meet RDA for vitamins/minerals |

## TABLE 4-6  Sampling of Enteral Products (Continued)

| Indication | Formula/Manufacturer[a] | Kilocalories/Volume (mL) to Meet 100% RDA[b] for Micronutrients |
|---|---|---|
| Diabetes/ hyperglycemia and promotion of normal bowel movement | DiabetiSource/Novartis | 1,500/1,500 |
| | Choice DM/Mead Johnson | 1,000/948 |
| | FiberSource/Novartis | 1,250/1,500 |
| | Glytrol/Nestle | 1,400/1,400 |
| | Glucerna/Ross | 1,422/1,422 |
| | Jevity/Ross | 1,246/1,321 |
| | Profiber/Sherwood Medical | 1,250/1,250 |
| | Ultracal/Mead Johnson | 1,113/1,180 |

[a]Manufacturer information: Sherwood Medical, St. Louis, MO 63103; Novartis Nutrition, Fremont, MI 47413; Ross Laboratories, Abbott Park, IL 60064; Mead Johnson Nutritionals, Evansville, IN 47721; Nutrition Medical, Minneapolis, MN 55442; Nestle Clinical Nutrition, Deerfield, IL 60015; and McGaw, Irvine, CA 92714.

[b]RDA indicates US Recommended Dietary Allowances.

clinician may need to alter formula choice as the patient's clinical, psychosocial, or economic status changes.

## INFUSION OPTIONS

Infusion methods for enteral nutrition include bolus, gravity, continuous, cyclic, pump infused, or closed systems. Bolus feedings are best tolerated when low-osmolality formulas of reasonable volume (<400 mL) are used. Risk of aspiration is an important consideration for any method of tube feeding, including bolus and pump controlled. To reduce the risk of aspiration, nasojejunal tubes are inserted, and an opening is made in the jejunum past the Treitz ligament. In a hospital setting, continuous feeding with enteral feeding pumps are generally used for patients with limited mobility and where accurate accounts of infused volume are required. Cyclic feedings are advantageous when attempting to make a transition from enteral nutrition to oral support and are implemented frequently on a nocturnal basis. Although controversial and not completely understood, night feeding may stimulate the appetite in some patients during the day or at least not suppress it, as might be expected (9). Cyclic feedings can be cumbersome in a hospital

## TABLE 4-7  Sampling of Modular Enteral Products

| Formula | Manufacturer[a] | Comments |
|---|---|---|
| Casec | Mead Johnson | Protein, 4.7 g/T, calcium caseinate |
| Elementra | Nestle | Protein, 4.5 g/T, whey |
| ProMod | Ross Products | Protein, 4 g/T, whey |
| Propac | Sherwood Medical | Protein, 4 g/T, whey |
| Moducal | Mead Johnson | Carbohydrate, 8 g/T, hydrolyzed cornstarch |
| Polycose | Ross Products | Carbohydrate, 6 g/T, hydrolyzed cornstarch |
| Sumacal | Sherwood Medical | Carbohydrate, 5 g/T, maltodextrin |
| MCT oil | Mead Johnson | Fat, MCT oil |
| Microlipid | Sherwood | Medical Fat, safflower oil with emulsifier |

[a]Manufacturer information: Mead Johnson Nutritionals, Evansville, IN 47721; Ross Laboratories, Abbott Park, IL 60064; and Sherwood Medical, St. Louis, MO 63103.

setting, where monitoring may be conducted by several different personnel shifts. Cyclic or intermittent feedings are also commonly instituted in the home care setting, as they allow greater flexibility for ambulatory patients.

A hang time of no more than 4 hours is recommended when enteral feeding is infused in an open system. Closed systems, requiring no mixing or filling of bags, have the unique advantages of bacterial safety and ease of administration (10). Although they have not gained widespread use in the hospital setting, where clinical needs are sometimes more dynamic, these products may be used more often in home care and long-term-care facilities for their convenience and safety features. New packaging technology, the "air-independent" enteral bag, allows the safety of a closed system and a greater flexibility for bolus and intermittent feedings.

## ENTERAL FEEDING TUBES

As with enteral formulas, there is a preponderance of enteral feeding tubes. Nonsurgical orogastric, nasoenteric, percutaneous endoscopic gastrostomy, surgically placed pharyngostomy, esophagostomy, and enterostomy are all routes that may be used. Short-term feedings in an institutional setting may be nasoenteric. Longer term feedings and tube feedings outside the institutional setting tend to be percutaneous endoscopically placed or surgically placed enterostomies. Low-profile gastrostomies are also considered for long-term feedings ($\geq 30$ days), ease of care, and cosmetic reasons. Some devices, such as nasally placed tubes, may be less suited to patients who have chronic coughing fits.

When deciding on the most appropriate tube to use, the clinician must consider four key factors: patient comfort, need for medication administration, cost, and site for infusion. Examples of tube categories are nasogastric, nasojejunal, percutaneous endoscopic gastrostomy, and percutaneous endoscopic jejunostomy. An appropriate choice of products is essential to the success of enteral feeding. The same considerations should be given for surgically placed tubes that are given for any other invasive procedures.

## EFFICACY OF ENTERAL SUPPORT

The use of enteral feeding to replenish the nutritional stores of malnourished HIV-infected patients appears to be effective. Several studies have demonstrated the ability to not only increase body weight but also improve serum albumin, total iron binding capacity, and total body potassium measures (3, 11). This seems to be achievable with short-term nutrition support of only 2 to 4 months' duration. Although CD4 cell counts have not improved with aggressive enteral support, improvement in several nutrition-related measures has been suggested (12). Nonresponders to enteral nutrition support, those patients who do not rehabilitate BCM, should be evaluated for alternate feeding methods and adjunctive support (2).

TABLE 4-8  Complications of Enteral Feeding and Interventions

| Complication | Solution |
| --- | --- |
| Diarrhea | Slow feeding rate; continuous feeding; increase or decrease fiber content; check for contamination; provide at room temperature; trial of peptide-based formula; avoid lactose; evaluate antidiarrheal medications, such as octreotide acetate (Sandostatin, Sandoz Pharmaceuticals, East Hanover, NJ 07936), deodorized tincture of opium, diphenoxylate hydrochloride with atropine sulfate (Lomotil, GD Searle, Chicago, IL 60680), and loperamide hydrochloride (Imodium, McNeil PPC, Fort Washington, PA 19034); avoid hypertonic medications |
| Constipation | Increase fluids; increase activity; physical therapy; provide fiber; maintain normal potassium levels; stool softeners |
| Aspiration | Feed into small intestine distal to the ligament of Treitz; keep head of bed elevated >30 degrees while feeding and 2 hours past infusion; reduce fat content of formula; try intermittent, small-volume feeding; avoid respiratory suction during feeding and check tube placement after any oral suctioning |
| Clogged feeding tube | Flush tubing with warm tap water; avoid cranberry juice or soda; check with pharmacist about medication administration via feeding tubes; substitute larger tube; avoid calorically dense or viscous formulas; clean and flush the tube system every 8-12 hours; shake hanging formula periodically and before initiating feeding; try pancreatic enzymes; try physical apparatuses available to unclog tubes |
| Nausea and distention | Continue feeding as tolerated; feed into small bowel; decrease osmolality with lower bowel feedings; slow administration rate; administer at room temperature; avoid lactose; evaluate medications; decrease fiber or fat content |
| Contamination | Use closed systems; use sterile water; decrease hang time; do not add old formula to new; practice good hand washing and infection control; discard open formula after 24 hours of refrigeration |
| Nasal irritation, necrosis | Use smallest bore tube possible; avoid use of nasogastric suction tubes for feeding; use flexible polyurethane tubes; avoid pressure points; use petroleum jelly on contact areas; use porous securing tape and the smallest amount necessary; tape loosely; consider conversion of feeding tube to percutaneous endoscopic gastrostomy or percutaneous endoscopic jejunostomy |

## COMPLICATIONS

The complications associated with enteral feeding are similar for both the general patient population and patients with HIV disease. Complications include diarrhea, constipation, aspiration, clogged feeding tube, nausea, gastrointestinal distention, nasal irritation, and contamination of the formula. Possible solutions to these complications are listed in Table 4-8. The issue of contamination takes on an increased significance for patients with HIV disease. Sterile preparation techniques and strict adherence to the manufacturer's suggested hang times are essential. The use of home or institutional blended formulas is discouraged.

Before a clinician crushes or dilutes medications, a pharmacist should be consulted. If medicines are administered through feeding tubes, they need to be flushed with water before and after administration. Sustained-release drugs, liquid-filled capsules, and enteric-coated medicines cannot be crushed for administration through feeding tubes (13). A pharmacist should also be asked about potential drug-nutrient interactions and clogging of tubes (14). Some medications are altered in terms of bioavailability and effectiveness. Therefore, close communication among the dietitian, pharmacist, and nurse about providing medications to patients on tube feeding is essential to the health care plan.

### MANAGEMENT AND MONITORING

The management and monitoring of enteral support should include a team approach. Team members may include the patient, physician, dietitian, pharmacist, nurse, social worker, psychologist, physical and occupational therapists, speech pathologist, and others. Use of a team approach is clearly cost-effective and ensures optimal nutrition care for the patient (15-18). Monitoring of the patient's clinical course, tolerance to feedings, changes in nutritional status, and biochemical values may be facilitated by accurate recording of flow sheets, which allow the team to identify trends and provide necessary intervention before problems escalate.

Dietitians should become comfortable with recommending necessary interventions to correct deficits or excesses of key nutrients, such as potassium, sodium, magnesium, chloride, glucose, vitamins and minerals, and trace elements. Many of these nutrients can be tracked by serum levels on a nutrition support flow sheet; others demonstrate an indirect relationship (eg, carbohydrate intake and its effect on serum glucose and triglyceride levels).

Weight and fluid status are other aspects of monitoring that are easily incorporated into flow sheets. A single weight or fluid intake and output may not be as relevant as trends documented over days. An example of an enteral flow sheet is shown in Figure 4-2. For most HIV-infected patients receiving nutrition support, the general and laboratory data can be safely monitored using the guidelines shown in Tables 4-9 and 4-10. As noted in Table 4-10, certain laboratory values, such as renal function tests, calcium, magnesium, and phosphorus, may need to be evaluated often during the initial phase of feeding.

Once metabolic stability is demonstrated, the frequency of monitoring may be decreased. Other laboratory data, such as albumin levels or the results of liver function tests, should be evaluated on a routine basis according to the patient's clinical fragility and the usability of laboratory values to adjust therapy.

## Parenteral Support

Parenteral nutrition (PN) support is defined as the provision of nutrients administered intravenously. Although nutrient provision is an important goal, it is second in importance to metabolic stabilization and main-

**FIGURE 4-2 Enteral Nutrition Monitoring Sheet**[a]

| Date | | | | | | | | | | |
|---|---|---|---|---|---|---|---|---|---|---|
| TF day # | | | | | | | | | | |
| Na+ | | | | | | | | | | |
| K+ | | | | | | | | | | |
| $CO_2$ | | | | | | | | | | |
| Glucose | | | | | | | | | | |
| BUN | | | | | | | | | | |
| Creatinine | | | | | | | | | | |
| Calcium | | | | | | | | | | |
| Phosphate | | | | | | | | | | |
| Mg+ | | | | | | | | | | |
| Albumin | | | | | | | | | | |
| Total Protein | | | | | | | | | | |
| Prealbumin | | | | | | | | | | |
| Total direct bilirubin | | | | | | | | | | |
| AST(SGOT) | | | | | | | | | | |
| Alkaline phosphates | | | | | | | | | | |
| ALT(SGPT) | | | | | | | | | | |
| Triglycerides | | | | | | | | | | |
| Amylase | | | | | | | | | | |
| Lipase | | | | | | | | | | |
| WBC | | | | | | | | | | |
| Hemoglobin | | | | | | | | | | |
| Hematocrit | | | | | | | | | | |
| Other | | | | | | | | | | |
| Enteral formula | | | | | | | | | | |
| Strength | | | | | | | | | | |
| Rate (mL/hr) | | | | | | | | | | |
| Kcal/d | | | | | | | | | | |
| protein/d | | | | | | | | | | |
| NPC:N | | | | | | | | | | |
| Oral intake | | | | | | | | | | |
| Other: IV, TPN | | | | | | | | | | |
| Weight | | | | | | | | | | |
| Intake | | | | | | | | | | |
| Output | | | | | | | | | | |
| Temperature | | | | | | | | | | |

Location:
Patient name:
Patient ID#:

Age:        M        F
DOB:
Admit date:
MD/Team:
Height:
Weight:
Goal weight:
Weight for calculation:

Enteral
Rate
kcal/d
kcal/kg per day
Protein g/d
g/kg

Diagnosis:

PMHx/surge

Allergies:

Medications:

Desired
Measures:

Outcome:
Oral

TPN
Withdraw NS

[a]TF indicates tube feeding; Na, sodium; K, potassium; $CO_2$, carbon dioxide; BUN, serum (blood) urea nitrogen; Mg, magnesium; AST, aspartate aminotransferase; ALT, alanine aminotransferase; WBC, white blood cell count; NPC:N, nonprotein calories to nitrogen ratio; IV, intravenous; TPN, total parenteral nutrition; DOB, date of birth; PMHx, past medical history; and NS, nutrition support.

TABLE 4-9  Nutrition Support Monitoring Categories

| Monitoring Category | Methods |
| --- | --- |
| Nutritional | Dietary intake, weight, serum protein levels, anthropometry when available/appropriate: nitrogen balance, bioelectrical impedance analysis |
| Metabolic | Electrolytes, mineral status (sodium, potassium, phosphorus, calcium, magnesium), glucose, and others |
| Gastrointestinal function | Change in bowel elimination, consistency, frequency; check gastric residual and/or gastrointestinal motility; check for suspected malabsorption with d-xylose test and/or fecal fat test |
| Mechanical | Tube placement/patency, skin integrity, raised head of bed, irrigation, dressing changes, tube/bag changes, and others |

tenance. The use of PN support is largely indicated based on meeting the nutrition needs of a patient with a nonfunctional or extremely compromised gastrointestinal tract. Parenteral nutrition support may be the most appropriate route for nutrition support of patients with HIV disease in the presence of the following conditions:

- AIDS enteropathy.
- Intractable emesis.
- Acute pancreatitis with pain and complications.
- Herpes simplex virus with ulcerative lesions of the perianal area or rectum.
- Infection with *Microsporidia* and *Cryptosporidium* species, cytomegalovirus (CMV) of the bowel, or *Mycobacterium avium-intracellulare* (MAI) of the gastrointestinal tract in combination with copious, persistent diarrhea.
- Intolerance of enteral support.

As much as possible, PN should not be used for patients who have functional gastrointestinal tracts. In severe cases, some patients may be too metabolically unstable to initiate nutrition support with the purpose of nutritional status rehabilitation. In these cases, PN may be initiated with the goal to metabolically stabilize a patient before nutritional reha-

TABLE 4-10  Laboratory Monitoring of HIV-Infected Patients Receiving Nutrition Support[a]

| Start-Up Laboratory Monitoring (Baseline Data) | Follow-Up Laboratory Monitoring |
| --- | --- |
| Albumin | Weekly |
| Prealbumin | Biweekly (every Monday and Thursday) |
| Calcium, magnesium, phosphorus | Biweekly (every Monday and Thursday) |
| Electrolytes, BUN, creatinine, glucose | Daily for 1 week |
| Complete blood cell counts | Biweekly (every Monday and Thursday) |
| Liver function tests | Weekly |
| Triglycerides | Biweekly |

[a]Frequency and specificity of monitoring will vary between patients, their clinical status, and health care setting.

bilitation. Patients who are responding to oral or enteral measures and would find the initiation of PN a setback should be encouraged to continue their course of therapy unless it is deemed contraindicated. In cases of terminal disease in which fluid and electrolyte replacement is the primary concern, intravenous (IV) fluids with electrolytes or even moderate protein load may be appropriately used depending on the patient's wishes.

In addition, patients receiving PN do not necessarily need to avoid oral intake. Enteral stimulation of the gut may be especially important in HIV disease to preserve gut integrity and immune function. In many cases the continued encouragement to consume nutrients orally, even in the presence of malabsorption, will promote self-care and patient control over an aspect of clinical care.

An understanding of the transitional feeding process as a marker of improvement can smooth the change to oral intake. However, in some cases, the use of combination therapies will affect reimbursement. For instance, Medicare may require PN to be the sole source of nutrients for more than 90 days to qualify for reimbursement as a medically necessary therapy. This stance may be especially detrimental to patients with HIV disease, since it may further compromise gut function.

## SELECTION OF A PARENTERAL ROUTE

Central and peripheral lines are the two routes used for PN support. Central or total PN (TPN) is infused via the jugular or subclavian veins in most instances. This route is generally used for longer term support (>7 days) or in patients with fluid or volume restriction, as with renal, cardiac, or hepatic failure (Figure 4-3). Furthermore, if peripheral access is poor, as with patients with a history of injection drug use, chemotherapy, or other multiple IV drug therapies, a central line must be used to reduce the risk of phlebitis. Central nutrition support may require surgical placement of the line or catheter. Indwelling catheters, such as the Hickman or Groshong, are frequently used when it is anticipated the patient will be discharged with the catheter in place. Alternately, peripherally inserted central catheters (PICC) have gained popularity because they do not require surgical placement by a physician and allow for easy care of the exit site by the patient. Antibiotic-coated PICC lines are available for patients with a history of, or at high risk for, line infection.

Peripheral PN (PPN) is administered through smaller veins, usually in the hand or lower arm, and generally used for a period less than 7 days. Peripheral nutrition support may be used as an adjunct to oral or enteral support or as a temporary feeding measure during bouts of pancreatitis or medical workup of malabsorptive syndromes. Patient education about the risks and benefits of various infusion sites is essential for patient decision-making.

Infection is of great concern in HIV disease. Patients need to be educated about its prevalence and the appropriate preventive measures to reduce risk for line sepsis. A well-trained patient may be able to appropriately administer PN therapy and care for catheters and other equipment involved. This process encourages self-care and supports the patient's ability to report any problems to the health care team.

**FIGURE 4-3  Feeding Route Decision Tree**

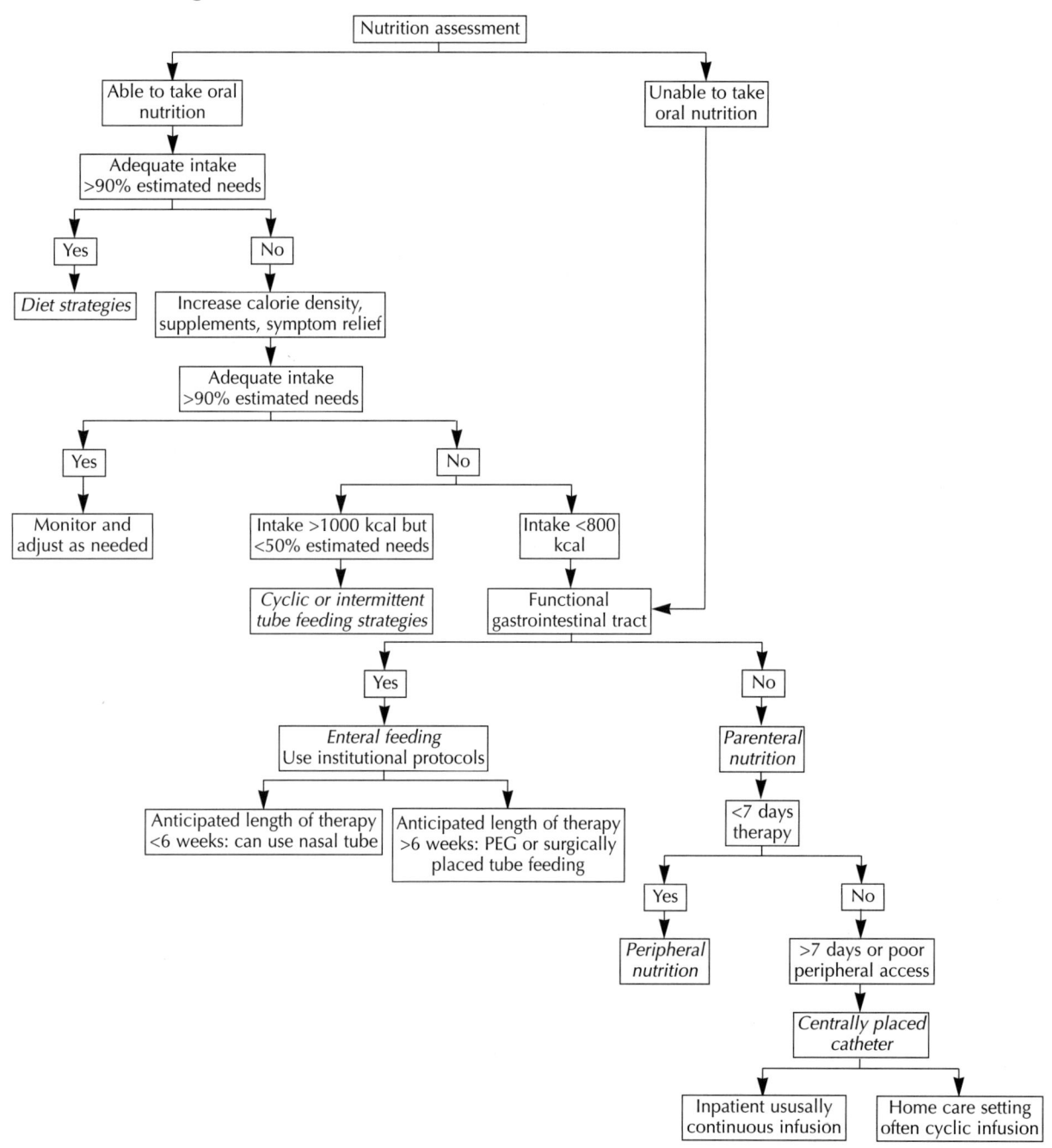

```
                          Nutrition assessment
                         /                    \
                Able to take              Unable to take
                oral nutrition            oral nutrition
                      |                         |
                Adequate intake                 |
                >90% estimated needs            |
                  /       \                     |
                Yes        No                   |
                 |          |                   |
            Diet         Increase calorie       |
            strategies   density, supplements,  |
                         symptom relief         |
                              |                 |
                         Adequate intake        |
                         >90% estimated needs   |
                          /        \            |
                        Yes         No          |
                         |           |          |
                    Monitor and    / \          |
                    adjust as    /    \         |
                    needed                      |
              Intake >1000 kcal but   Intake <800 kcal
              <50% estimated needs           |
                      |                      |
              Cyclic or intermittent    Functional  <—
              tube feeding strategies   gastrointestinal tract
                                          /        \
                                        Yes         No
                                         |           |
                                  Enteral feeding   Parenteral
                                  Use institutional  nutrition
                                  protocols             |
                                   /       \        <7 days
                          Anticipated   Anticipated  therapy
                          length of     length of    /    \
                          therapy       therapy    Yes    No
                          <6 weeks:     >6 weeks:   |      |
                          can use       PEG or    Peripheral  >7 days or poor
                          nasal tube    surgically nutrition  peripheral access
                                        placed                     |
                                        tube feeding         Centrally placed
                                                             catheter
                                                              /        \
                                                     Inpatient      Home care setting
                                                     ususally       often cyclic infusion
                                                     continuous
                                                     infusion
```

PEG indicates percutaneous endoscopic gastrostomy.

## PARENTERAL NUTRITION SOLUTIONS

To calculate the most appropriate base solution for PN, the following must be considered: the infusion route (central vs peripheral), nutrient requirements of the patient, presence of biochemical abnormalities (especially in relation to glucose, lipid, or amino acid intolerance), plans for future cyclic or home PN support, and medications prescribed. The concentration and quantity of protein, lipid, and dextrose, as well as supplemental micronutrients beyond standard additives, will be individualized.

Regimens of TPN are commonly dextrose based. Dextrose-based solutions are generally well tolerated in the HIV population as long as the dextrose load is less than 5 mg/kg/minute. Since HIV disease is a chronic inflammatory disease and some level of metabolic stress may be assumed, prudent calculation of dextrose load may be at levels of 4 to 5 mg/kg actual body weight per minute (4 to 5 mg/kg/minute). The maximum dose within a safe range is 5 mg. For the patient in the home care setting or receiving cyclic TPN, it is crucial to include safe levels of dextrose infusion as a part of patient education.

Patients who are HIV infected may demonstrate an intolerance to lipids by an elevation in serum triglyceride levels. However, there is not necessarily a concomitant rise in serum triglyceride levels in HIV-infected patients receiving IV lipids. Therefore, levels need to be monitored. A baseline elevation in triglyceride levels should not preclude use of IV lipids unless postinfusion levels approach extremely elevated levels compared with baseline measurements. Triglyceride levels are often elevated in HIV disease, and a change may indicate an acute phase of infection rather than lipid intolerance (19). Lipid levels should be checked 1 to 2 hours after infusion for more accurate results. During continuous infusion of lipids, blood samples can be drawn on the alternate arm for analysis of triglyceride levels. In addition, some data suggest that IV lipids may increase the prevalence of infections and sepsis when kilocalories from lipid comprise greater than 35% of the total kilocalories infused (16). This remains controversial, but it is prudent to use a lower level of lipid in HIV-infected patients than in patients with normal immune function. The percent energy contribution in peripheral PN may be greater. In general, maximum load recommendations are at the level of 1 g/kg/day or less, which translates to 5 mL of 20% lipid or 10 mL of 10% lipid per kilogram per day.

The use of 3-in-1 admixture (a combination of dextrose, amino acids, and lipids) is a widely accepted practice in most patient populations, including HIV disease. However, a 3-in-1 admixture may make a filtering process difficult due to the size of lipid molecules. A contraindication to the use of a 3-in-1 formulation would be in cases where the necessary level of additives to achieve nutrient requirements is high enough to risk the formation of a precipitate that may not be filtered in a 3-in-1 solution.

## MICRONUTRIENTS

Before initiating support, baseline laboratory values should be evaluated. Measurements taken after initiation of nutrition support and serially will help to monitor metabolic processes and tolerance to feeding regimens. Table 4-11 offers a composite of micronutrient supplementation guidelines for adults receiving PN support.

## ELECTROLYTES

Fluid and electrolytes are critical parameters to monitor in patients with HIV disease. Potassium, magnesium, phosphorus, and sodium levels often need to be supplemented, especially in cases of diarrhea or fever. If additional fluid provision is indicated, it may be appropriate to give fluids separately from the TPN or as a piggyback, especially since TPN is routinely billed by the liter; therefore, expanding TPN volume to meet fluid requirements may not be cost-effective. Several medications can also increase electrolyte requirements as indicated earlier, and in these cases additional replacement therapy likely will be needed.

Severe hypophosphatemia frequently accompanies the "refeeding syndrome," which is characterized by sudden cardiopulmonary failure in chronically malnourished HIV-infected patients who receive aggressive nutrition support (9). Patients with HIV may be at risk of the refeeding syndrome if acute, severe weight loss occurs before parenteral feeding. Phosphorus, potassium, and magnesium levels should be aggressively replaced and monitored. Standard parenteral levels of these nutrients will likely need to be increased to 1.25 to 1.5 times standard levels to maintain stores during the first 1 to 2 weeks of support (16). Levels higher than twice the normal values may result in undesirable precipitation; therefore, any correction or supplementation above this level

**TABLE 4-11   Micronutrient Requirements of Patients Receiving Parenteral Nutrition Support**

| Vitamin/Trace Element | Recommended Intake for Adults |
|---|---|
| Vitamin A (IU) | 4,000-5,000 |
| Vitamin D (IU) | 400 |
| Vitamin E (IU) | 12-15 |
| Vitamin C (mg) | 60 |
| Niacin (mg) | 12-20 |
| Riboflavin (mg) | 1.1-1.8 |
| Thiamin (mg) | 1-1.5 |
| Pyridoxine (mg) | 1.6-2 |
| Pantothenic acid (mg) | 5-10 |
| Folic acid (μg) | 400 |
| Biotin (μg) | 100-300 |
| Vitamin B-12 (μg) | 3 |
| Copper (mg) | 0.5-1.5 |
| Chromium (μg) | 10-15 |
| Iron (mg) | — |
| Manganese (mg) | 0.15-0.8 |
| Zinc (mg) | 2.5-4 |

should be given via a separate IV bolus. If phosphorus levels are below 1.2, magnesium below 1, or potassium below 3, aggressive replacement with IV therapy is indicated. Parenteral iron supplements should be avoided unless necessary, since increased levels of iron may increase susceptibility to infection even in the presence of low serum iron levels. In addition, IV iron can result in an anaphylactic reaction in some individuals.

## TRACE ELEMENTS

Limited data are available on the trace element requirements of HIV-positive patients. It appears there may be a tendency toward deficiencies of copper, selenium, and zinc. These micronutrients may be supplemented at a level 1.5 to 2 times the usual recommended dosage (16). Several trace element preparations include selenium and can be administered daily with TPN. If these preparations do not include selenium, a dose of 0.87 µg/kg/day is recommended, especially if TPN has been administered for more than 20 days. Parenteral zinc replacement (2.5 to 4 mg) is necessary in patients with excessive losses due to diarrhea, fistulas, or open wounds; excessive replacement is not advised, as it may suppress immune function (16, 20, 21).

## VITAMINS

Standard parenteral vitamin supplementation for HIV-infected patients should follow the clinician's institutional or agency guidelines. In cases of diarrhea, additional water-soluble vitamin replacement (twice normal) is indicated. Folate, B-12, B-6, thiamin, and vitamin C supplementation at twice the normal levels have been recommended, because altered levels in these vitamins are commonly identified in this patient population (4). Special care should be taken with administration of all nutrients to prevent precipitation, interactions with drug therapies, overfeeding and toxic levels of micronutrients, and metabolic instability.

## COMPLICATIONS OF PARENTERAL NUTRITION

Catheter-related problems and sepsis are the two major complications associated with PN. Catheter-related complications may stem from the technique used or lack of experience by the clinician placing the line. Such complications include pneumothorax, hydrothorax, or chylothorax, subclavian artery puncture, subclavian vein thrombosis, air emboli, or malposition of the catheter (22).

Sepsis is a potentially life-threatening complication. It is diagnosed when a microorganism is isolated from the catheter tip and is also found in the patient's blood. *Staphylococcus aureus* and *Candida* species are the most common pathogens for catheter-related sepsis. HIV infection is a major risk factor for developing catheter-related sepsis. Rates of infection associated with Hickman catheters in patients with AIDS were 0.47 in one study and 0.17 in another, both per 100 catheter days (23, 24). A third study documented a significant difference in infection rates between HIV-infected patients and other patients receiving TPN, and again this was in association with the use of Hickman catheters (25).

Infection may be avoided by maintaining proper sterile mixing and handling of solutions and by following infection control procedures (see the next section). Additionally, it is advisable to reduce manipulation of the catheter as much as possible; the literature on catheter-related sepsis has found a close association between the incidence of infection and the frequency of catheter manipulation (26). Antibiotic treatment before and after insertion of a catheter also is recommended to prevent an infection. If an infection develops, the catheter should be removed (23, 24). Clinical signs of resolution of the infection (reduced fever, improved glucose tolerance, reduced white blood cell count, and normalized heart rate) typically occur with removal of the catheter.

In deciding whether to use PN, the clinician should take into account the patient's nutritional status and ability to mount an inflammatory response to catheter infection. An extremely wasted patient may not show signs of serious infection until nutritional repletion begins. The consequences of infection in an immunocompromised patient are far more serious than with the general patient population; therefore, close monitoring for early detection and intervention is critical.

## INFECTION CONTROL

Infection control is important for both the patient and health care professional. Most health care institutions and agencies have adopted universal precautions aimed at preventing transmission of communicable diseases, such as hepatitis or HIV. These consist of standard activities surrounding patient care and handling of medical equipment, as listed below (27):

1. Thoroughly wash your hands with soap and water before and after working with patients. Wear gloves and protective clothing (lab coats or smocks) when working with open wounds or other lesions, or in any case when contact with blood or bodily fluids is likely.
2. Carefully clean surfaces with appropriate cleaning solutions and sprays when they are soiled by bodily fluids.
3. Dispose of supplies in heavy plastic bags or double bags according to community disposal guidelines and regulations. Needles ("sharps") should be disposed of in puncture-proof containers. Disinfect nondisposable items with a 10% bleach solution.

At home or in nonmedical situations, additional precautions should become routine. Washing dishes, laundry, and other household cleaning in regular soap or other cleansing agent and water should be sufficient; durable medical equipment should be cleaned with a 10% bleach solution (such as glucometers) (27).

## MANAGEMENT AND MONITORING

Monitoring of PN is essential for three reasons. First, monitoring helps avoid metabolic complications, especially in the area of biochemical regulation. Second, it allows the clinician to continually evaluate and assess the nutritional status of the patient and the efficacy of the care provided. Third, monitoring can identify microbial complications associated with line sepsis. Table 4-3 outlines some of the most common biochemical alterations and causes. The use of flow sheets to monitor the clinical, biochemical, and nutritional parameters of the patient is essential (Figure 4-4).

The complications of overfeeding are of special concern. If a metabolic cart is available, close monitoring to maintain a respiratory quotient below 1 is recommended, especially with patients who have a history of respiratory insufficiency or chronic obstructive pulmonary disease. Overfeeding of kilocalories may contribute to respiratory distress in patients with opportunistic pneumonias and acid-base disorders, with the additional risk of organ dysfunction in the presence of renal insufficiency. For this and other reasons, the initial TPN solution may be calculated on minimum energy requirements and advanced with close monitoring, with priority given to metabolic stability over nutritional repletion.

## EFFICACY OF PARENTERAL NUTRITION SUPPORT

Reversing malnutrition with PN clearly indicates that repletion of visceral protein stores will have to occur during clinically stable periods. As with other acutely or critically ill patients, catabolic HIV-infected patients do not demonstrate reversal of these deficits. Rehabilitation of somatic protein stores may require physical activity and the normalization of protein synthesis vs lipid synthesis in the liver. Anecdotal reports of TPN in home care seem to support improved functional status and return to activities of daily living. Since rehabilitation is difficult at best with HIV-infected patients, the most beneficial and cost-effective use of TPN may be preventive, intermittent, and short term during early stages, when prevention of opportunistic infections and rehabilitation are more likely.

## TEAM APPROACH

For effective and efficient PN administration, a team approach to care is imperative. The team should at minimum consist of the patient, physician, clinical dietitian, clinical pharmacist, and nurse. A multidisciplinary team offers knowledge, resources, and support that are critical to the care of the patient, and it ensures that all team members make appropriate and consistent recommendations. A team approach can reduce both cost and complications of PN (16-18, 28).

# Role of the Registered Dietitian

Dietitians play an important role in ensuring the safe and effective use of enteral and PN support. They should be able to not only calculate the patients' nutritional requirements but also suggest specific changes in formulations when abnormal trends or laboratory values occur. For example, persistent hyperglycemia may trigger a recommendation for

**FIGURE 4-4  TPN Monitoring Sheet**

| | | | | | | | | | | | |
|---|---|---|---|---|---|---|---|---|---|---|---|
| Date | | | | | | | | | | | Location: |
| TPN day # | | | | | | | | | | | Patient name: |
| Na+ | | | | | | | | | | | Patient ID#: |
| K+ | | | | | | | | | | | |
| $CO_2$ | | | | | | | | | | | |
| Glucose | | | | | | | | | | | Age:    M    F |
| BUN | | | | | | | | | | | DOB: |
| Creatinine | | | | | | | | | | | Admit date: |
| Calcium | | | | | | | | | | | MD/Team: |
| Phosphate | | | | | | | | | | | Height: |
| Mg+ | | | | | | | | | | | Weight: |
| Albumin | | | | | | | | | | | Goal weight: |
| Total Protein | | | | | | | | | | | Weight for calculation: |
| Prealbumin | | | | | | | | | | | |
| Total direct bilirubin | | | | | | | | | | | TPN |
| AST(SGOT) | | | | | | | | | | | Rate |
| Alkaline phosphates | | | | | | | | | | | kcal/d |
| ALT(SGPT) | | | | | | | | | | | kcal/kg per day |
| Triglycerides | | | | | | | | | | | Protein g/d |
| Amylase | | | | | | | | | | | g/kg |
| Lipase | | | | | | | | | | | |
| WBC | | | | | | | | | | | Diagnosis: |
| Hemoglobin | | | | | | | | | | | |
| Hematocrit | | | | | | | | | | | |
| Platelets | | | | | | | | | | | PMHx/surge |
| PT/INR | | | | | | | | | | | |
| PTT | | | | | | | | | | | |
| Weight | | | | | | | | | | | |
| Intake | | | | | | | | | | | Allergies: |
| Output | | | | | | | | | | | |
| Temperature | | | | | | | | | | | Medications: |
| TPN Formula | | | | | | | | | | | |
| Rate (mL/hr) | | | | | | | | | | | |
| Dextrose (final) | | | | | | | | | | | |
| Amino Acids (final) | | | | | | | | | | | |
| Fat (final) | | | | | | | | | | | |
| NaCl (mEq/L) | | | | | | | | | | | |
| K as phosphate (mEq/L) | | | | | | | | | | | |
| KCl (mEq/L) | | | | | | | | | | | |
| Mg sulfate (mEq/L) | | | | | | | | | | | |
| Ca gluconate (mEq/L) | | | | | | | | | | | |
| MVI-12 | | | | | | | | | | | |
| Trace elements | | | | | | | | | | | |
| Type/amount | | | | | | | | | | | |
| Phytonadoine (mg/L) | | | | | | | | | | | Desired |
| Heparin (U/L) | | | | | | | | | | | Measures: |
| Folic acid (mg/L) | | | | | | | | | | | Outcome: |
| Ascorbic acid (mg/L) | | | | | | | | | | | Oral |
| Regular insulin (U/L) | | | | | | | | | | | Tube feed |
| K acetate (mEq/L) | | | | | | | | | | | Withdraw NS |
| Na acetate (mEq/L) | | | | | | | | | | | |
| Zinc (mg/L) | | | | | | | | | | | |
| K-runs (mEq) | | | | | | | | | | | |
| Mg supplement | | | | | | | | | | | |
| FS/SS insulin | | | | | | | | | | | |
| ABGs: pH | | | | | | | | | | | |
| $PCO_2/HCO_3$ | | | | | | | | | | | |

[a]TPN indicates total parenteral nutrition; Na, sodium; K, potassium; $CO_2$, carbon dioxide; BUN, serum (blood) urea nitrogen; Mg, magnesium; AST, aspartate aminotransferase; ALT, alanine aminotransferase; WBC, white blood cell count; PT/INR, prothrombin time/international normalization ratio; PTT, partial thromboplastin time; NaCl, sodium chloride; Ca, calcium; DOB, date of birth; PMHx, past medical history; FS/SS, fingerstick sugar/serum sugar; ABGs, arterial blood gases; $PCO_2/HCO_3$, carbon dioxide partial pressure/bicarbonate; and NS, nutrition support.

the reduction of dextrose load and the provision of additional lipid to replace lost dextrose kilocalories. Or, if a patient demonstrates ongoing hypomagnesemia, the dietitian may recommend necessary increases in the TPN magnesium level to replace losses and correct the deficit. A foundation of knowledge in the evaluation and treatment of acid-base balance is essential to the safe use of TPN. Dietitians should also provide patient education about signs and symptoms for monitoring the safety and efficacy of PN outside an institutional setting. Team discussion is essential to determine the appropriateness of recommendations and their successful implementation.

## Summary

The identification and provision of appropriate care to candidates for specialized nutrition support can improve the quality of life and perhaps length of life for persons with HIV disease. The recommendations for successful specialized nutrition support in HIV present an exciting challenge to clinicians. Interventions should be individualized and provided as early as deemed appropriate by a multidisciplinary team, with input from the patient and concerned family members.

### References

1. Yeoh D, Lin HC. Nutritional support in patients with AIDS. *Nutr Notes.* 1995;7:1-2.
2. Hellerstein MK, Kahn J, Mudie H, Viteri F. Current approach to the treatment of human immunodeficiency virus associated weight loss: pathophysiologic considerations and emerging management strategies. *Semin Oncol.* 1990;17(suppl 9):17-33.
3. Kotler DP, Tierney AR, Culpepper JA, Wang J, Pierson RN. Effect of home total parenteral nutrition upon body composition in AIDS. *JPEN.* 1990;14:454-458.
4. Bogden JD, Baker H, Frank O, Perez G, Kemp F, Bruening K, Louria D. Micronutrient status and human immunodeficiency virus (HIV) infection. *Ann NY Acad Sci.* 1990;587:189-195.
5. Coodley GO, Coodley MK, Nelson HD, Loveless MO. Micronutrient concentrations in the HIV wasting syndrome. *AIDS.* 1993;7:1595-1600.
6. Beach RS, Mantero-Atienza E, Shor-Posner G, Javier GH, Szapocznik J, Morgan R, Sauberlich HE, Cornwell PE, Eisdorfer C, Baum MK. Specific nutrient abnormalities in asymptomatic HIV-1 infection. *AIDS.* 1992;6:701-708.
7. Abrams B, Duncan D, Hertz-Picciotto I. A prospective study of dietary intake and acquired immune deficiency syndrome in HIV-seropositive homosexual men. *J AIDS.* 1993;6:949-958.
8. Tang AM, Graham NMH, Kirby AJ, McCall LC, Willett WC, Saah AJ. Dietary micronutrient intake and risk of progression to human immunodeficiency virus type 1 (HIV-1)-infected homosexual men. *Am J Epidemiol.*1993;138:937-951.
9. Skipper A. *Dietitian's Handbook of Enteral and Parenteral Nutrition.* Gaithersburg, Md: Aspen Publishers; 1989.
10. Vaughan L, Manore M, Wilson D. Bacterial safety of a closed-administration system for enteral nutrition. *J Am Diet Assoc.* 1988;88:35-37.
11. Kotler DP, Tierney AR, Ferraro R, Cuff P, Wang J, Pierson RN, Heymsfeld SB. Enteral alimentation and repletion of body cell mass in malnourished patients with acquired immunodeficiency syndrome. *Am J Clin Nutr.* 1991;53:149-154.
12. Grunfeld C, Kotler DP. The wasting syndrome and nutritional support in AIDS. *Semin Gastrointest Dis.* 1991;2:25-36.
13. The Chicago Dietetic Association and The South Suburban Dietetic Association. *Manual of Clinical Dietetics*, 5th ed. Chicago, Ill: American Dietetic Association; 1996:320.

14. Lehmann S. Medication administration via feeding tubes. In: Teasley-Strausburg KM, ed. *Nutrition Support Handbook: A Compendium of Products with Guidelines for Usage.* Cincinnati, Ohio: Harvey Whitney Books; 1992:307-315.
15. Lenzi MA. The nutrition support team: surviving and thriving in an era of reform. *Nutr Clin Pract.* 1994;9:226-232.
16. Rollins CJ. *Total Parenteral Nutrition: Preparation and Patient Monitoring.* Tucson: Arizona Pharmacy Society; 1986.
17. Gales BJ, Gales, MJ. Nutritional support teams: a review of comparative trials. *Ann Pharmacother.* 1994;28:227-35.
18. Maurer J, Weinbaum F, Turner J, Brady T, Pistone B, D'Addario V, Lun W, Ghazali B. Reducing the inappropriate use of parenteral nutrition in an acute care teaching hospital. *JEPN.* 1996;20:272-274.
19. Grunfeld C, Feingold KR. The role of the cytokines, interferon alpha and tumor necrosis factor in the hypertriglyceridemia and wasting of AIDS. *J Nutr.* 1992;122(suppl):749-753.
20. Chandra RK. Nutrition, immunity, and infection: present knowledge and future directions. *Lancet.* 1983;1:688-691.
21. Baumgartner TG, ed. *Clinical Guide to Parenteral Micronutrition.* Melrose Park, IL: Educational Publications; 1984.
22. Moorwessel M, Hopkins B, Buzby KM. Human immunodeficiency virus infection. In: Gottschlich MM, Matarese LE, Shronts EP, eds. *Nutrition Support Dietetics.* 2nd ed. Silver Spring, Md: American Society for Parenteral and Enteral Nutrition; 1993:261-275.
23. Raviglione MC, Battan R, Pablos-Mendez A, Aceves-Casillas P, Mullen MP, Taranta A. Infections associated with Hickman catheters in patients with acquired immunodeficiency syndrome. *Am J Med.* 1989;86:780-786.
24. Mukau L, Talamini MA, Sitzman JV, Burns RC, McGuire ME. Long-term central venous access vs other home therapies: complications in patients with immunodeficiency syndrome. *JPEN.* 1992;16:455-459.
25. Tanner AG, Schellenberg D, Main J, Monson JR. A comparison between arm implanted (PASport), chest implanted (Port-A-Cath) and externally sited catheters (Hickman line) for long term venous access in AIDS patients. *Int Conf AIDS.* 1993;9(1):463. (abstract PoB25-1965).
26. Campbell SW, Lucas A. Implanted ports vs external catheters: infection rates of venous access devices in the treatment of CMV retinitis in AIDS patients. *Int Conf AIDS.* 1992;8:B133. Abstract PoB3280.
27. Visiting Nurses and Hospice of San Francisco. *AIDS Home Care and Hospice Manual.* San Francisco, Calif: Visiting Nurses and Hospice of San Francisco; 1987.
28. Hassell JT, Games AD, Shaffer B, Harkins LE. Nutrition support team management of enterally fed patients in a community hospital is cost-beneficial. *J Am Diet Assoc.* 1994;94:993-998.

# 5
# Assessment and Intervention Issues in Various Health Care Settings

The health care setting is one of four factors that the dietitian needs to consider in developing a nutrition care plan for persons with the human immunodeficiency virus (HIV) and the acquired immunodeficiency syndrome (AIDS). Other considerations that The American Dietetic Association and The Canadian Dietetic Association deem necessary in formulating this plan include the feasibility of reversing malnutrition, the patient's prognosis and motivation, and the proposed medical treatment goal (1). Where nutrition care is provided in different settings (acute- or long-term-care facility, outpatient clinic, home, community-based agency, or hospice) determines the appropriate approaches to resolving problems. The health care setting also affects how nutritional status is assessed, whether it is the dietitian and nurse keeping a calorie count in an institutional setting or the patient recording a food diary at home. Sometimes the choice of a health care service among patients is a matter of resources and economic feasibility.

## Inpatient Setting
### QUALITY OF CARE

Nutrition services as part of acute- and long-term care offer an opportunity to evaluate and monitor patients in a controlled setting. Patient medical records and nutrition care plans as well as dietitian's records and files are important sources of data that can be collected to assess the quality of care.

Bedside rounds are another means of gathering important information about the patient from a variety of professional perspectives. Patient rounds allow health care professionals to communicate as a team. Members of this team usually include the physician, nurse, clinical dietitian, clinical pharmacist, social worker, and perhaps a respiratory therapist and psychiatrist. Interacting with these colleagues at meetings or making notes in the patient's medical record provides an opportunity for dietitians to communicate their knowledge about current nutrition practices.

Teamwork can be illustrated in the following scenario. The addition of medical nutrition therapy can support the patient's recovery from opportunistic infections, improve response to therapies, and prevent serious wasting. In turn, the pharmacist can recommend a medication to improve the patient's appetite, the physician can write the prescription and discuss effective treatment strategies against *Pneumocystis carinii* pneumonia (PCP), the nurse can explain the treatment strategies to the patient, and all team members act as patient advocates (2). Later the dietitian monitors the patient's dietary intake and measures his or her body weight and triceps skinfold (TSF) thickness. The patient understands the treatment goals, starts to eat more, better tolerates medications, and recovers from PCP. Thus, teamwork benefits the patient.

The needs of the patient with HIV and the type of health care facility can dictate the length of stay from a few hours to several weeks. With budgetary cutbacks and cost containment, efforts are targeted at reducing the length of stay in acute-care settings. Therefore, dietitians need to be especially efficient in assessing and managing the nutrition care of patients.

Monitoring the quality of nutrition care in hospitals is a continuous process. One model developed for this purpose is based on continuous quality improvement concepts of the Joint Commission on Accreditation of Healthcare Organizations (JCAHO) (3). The concepts have been incorporated into the Yale-New Haven Hospital Nutritional Classification and Assessment Program (3). Although the program is not disease specific, there are practice guidelines in the model that could apply to patients with HIV. Examples follow:

- The patient has protein-energy malnutrition or is in the high-risk category for this condition. An oral diet has been ordered. A desirable outcome is to improve or stabilize nutritional status. The dietitian following these guidelines needs to conduct a thorough nutrition assessment (see Chapter 2) within 7 days of admission and to provide nutrition education as needed.
- The patient has protein-energy malnutrition and either needs or is receiving enteral nutrition or total parenteral nutrition. Two expected outcomes are to stabilize the metabolic or nutritional status and to prevent or reverse the catabolic state. The nutrition assessment should be carried out within 4 days of admission. Instructions about tube feedings or other pertinent dietary issues are provided to the patient and his or her caregiver before discharge.
- The patient has protein-energy malnutrition and is terminally ill. In this situation, the dietitian respects the preferences of the patient and the patient's family or caretaker. No formal nutrition education is required, although ongoing communication is important to clarify choices. Comfort foods that the patient can tolerate are provided.

This protocol used in the Yale-New Haven Hospital dictates that all patients whose length of stay in the hospital exceeds 3 days should be screened to determine if protein-energy malnutrition is present (3).

Ordinarily, a general nutrition screening, which includes diet prescription and general questions about dietary intake or appetite, is first used in a hospital by a nurse when the patient is admitted to the unit. If a certain number of risk factors for malnutrition are present, as specified individually by each hospital or clinical dietetics department, a patient may be referred to a dietitian for assessment (4). Figure 5-1 presents nutrition care standards for accrediting hospitals from the JCAHO. Based on the results of the nutrition screening and assessment (and ongoing reassessment if the patient is at nutritional risk), a nutrition care plan is developed. For inpatients with HIV, most of whom *are* at nutritional risk, measurable goals and a strategy to attain these goals make up the nutrition care plan.

## NUTRITION INTERVENTION

Nutrition intervention should start as soon as HIV disease is diagnosed. In the asymptomatic stage of HIV infection, the dietitian can emphasize the importance of eating a healthy, well-balanced diet rich in protein, energy, vitamins, and minerals. The objective is to teach the patient about the link between eating well and preserving weight and body cell mass. The fewer dietary changes the patient needs to make to meet nutrition goals, the more likely that the recommendations will be followed (5). In the patient with symptoms such as weight loss or infection, high-energy, nutrient-dense foods are often recommended, but the diet will probably need to be modified periodically (5). For example, a

---

**FIGURE 5-1  Nutrition Care Standards for JCAHO[a] Accreditation in Hospitals**

| | |
|---|---|
| TX.4. | Each patient's nutrition care is planned |
| TX.4.1. | An interdisciplinary nutrition therapy plan is developed and periodically updated for patients at nutritional risk |
| TX.4.1.1. | When appropriate to the patient groups served by a unit, meals and snacks support program goals |
| TX.4.2. | Authorized individuals prescribe or order food and nutrition products in a timely manner |
| TX.4.3. | Responsibilities are assigned for all activities involved in safe and accurate provision of food and nutrition products |
| TX.4.4. | Food and nutrition products are distributed and administered in a safe, accurate, timely, and acceptable manner |
| TX.4.5. | Each patient's response to nutrition care is monitored |
| TX.4.6. | The nutrition care service meets patients' needs for special diets and accommodates altered diet schedules |
| TX.4.7. | Nutrition care practices are standardized throughout the organization |

Source: *Comprehensive Accreditation Manual for Hospitals, 1997-98.* Oakbrook Terrace, Ill: Joint Commission on Accreditation of Health Care Organizations; 1996. (TX 29-33) Reprinted with permission.
[a]JCAHO indicates Joint Commission on Accreditation of Healthcare Organizations.

pureed or mechanical soft diet may be necessary for patients who have odynophagia or dysphagia (Table 5-1). If a calorie count shows that the patient's dietary intake is insufficient to reverse wasting, high-energy oral supplements and snacks should be served.

Later, enteral and parenteral nutrition options will need to be explored if the patient's condition deteriorates. Adequate discharge communication of the care plan to personnel in supervening settings is

**TABLE 5-1  Guidelines for Modifying the Content and Consistency of Foods for Patients With AIDS**

| Content/Consistency | Restriction/Modification | Indication |
|---|---|---|
| **Content** | | |
| Acid | Tomatoes, tomato sauce, vinegar, citrus fruits (oranges, grapefruits, lemons, limes), pineapples | Mouth pain due to oral or esophageal ulcers and thrush, gastric or intestinal ulcers, mouth sores from herpes, Kaposi's sarcoma lesions |
| Bland | All herbs and spices, peppers, chili powder, caffeine, salt, onion, garlic, vinegar | Mouth pain due to sores; oral, esophageal, or gastric ulcers; gastroesophageal reflux; nausea |
| Dairy | Milk, cheese, yogurt, ice cream, cream soups, sour cream, chocolate, butter, margarine, cottage cheese | Lactose intolerance, diarrhea |
| Fat (less than 20% total kilocalories) | Butter, whole-milk cheese, whole milk, nuts, fatty meats, poultry skin, fried food, oils, gravies, salad dressings, cream, cream soups, chocolate, mayonnaise, desserts made with shortening, avocados, olives | Diarrhea from fat malabsorption, nausea, pancreatitis, short-bowel syndrome |
| Fiber/gas (low residue/ low insoluble fiber) | Raw fruits, raw vegetables, broccoli, cabbage, cauliflower, peas, brussels sprouts, turnips, corn, whole grains, nuts, olives, onions, dried fruits, tough fibrous meats, peanut butter, beans | Diarrhea, flatulence, colitis, diverticulitis |
| Salt | Table salt, celery salt, garlic salt, monosodium glutamate, canned or salted meat, smoked meat or fish, frankfurters, ham bacon, kosher meats, luncheon meats, sausages, canned soups or any kind of commercial bouillon, canned vegetables or juices, dry cereals, processed cheese, olives, pickles, relishes, soy sauce, catsup | Edema/ascites, renal disease, liver disease, hypertension, heart failure |
| Sugar | Added sugar, concentrated sweets, chocolate, ice cream, sherbet, gelatin, soda, cakes and pastries containing sucrose, honey, catsup, carob powder, jams, jellies, corn syrup, molasses | Diabetes, glucose intolerance secondary to medications |
| **Consistency** | | |
| Soft | Most raw fruits and vegetables, very coarse breads and cereals, tough fibrous meats | Mouth pain due to oral or esophageal sores, difficult or painful swallowing |
| Minced | Food is chopped into finely sized pieces | Difficult swallowing, chewing difficulties or dental problems, aspiration |

Source: Abdale F. *Community-Based Nutrition Support for People Living With HIV and AIDS: A Technical Assistance Manual.* New York, NY: God's Love We Deliver; 1995. Used with permission.

crucial to the continuity of care and well-being of the patient. See Figure 5-2 for a sample discharge communication form.

### CLINICAL TRIALS FOR AIDS

Some dietitians are involved in clinical trials for HIV and HIV-related infections. Most of these trials evaluate wasting and experimental drugs and other therapies for adults and children at all stages of HIV infection. Appendix D provides a resource for more information on clinical trials.

## Outpatient and Clinic Settings

Formalized nutrition services in the clinic and outpatient departments of hospitals offer an opportunity to screen and evaluate patients in an ambulatory setting. The HIV-knowledgeable dietitian can provide screening tools for patients or health care personnel to complete. Criteria for referral may be included in the patient screening, or a separate screening tool may be available for a dietitian's review and recommendation for referral as needed (see Chapter 2). In clinics and other outpatient department settings, nutrition services may be provided on a referral-only basis or according to a clinic protocol. In either case, the dietitian can equip their referral sources with referral criteria and screening tools to use as needed (see Figure 5-3 for a sample referral format).

In many outpatient settings the medical record will be available for review by a dietitian. However, in some settings medical records may be less accessible. Adequate review of assessment criteria is crucial to develop appropriate and integrated care plans. Suggested standards of nutrition care for the outpatient clinic setting are shown in Figure 5-4. Documentation of evaluation and recommendations should be forwarded to the referral source and/or primary care physician. Communication methods should be established in advance to provide feedback to referring physicians to aid them in their responsibilities for coordinating patient care.

In addition to individualized evaluation, the outpatient setting may lend itself to providing group education on topics such as dietary hints to promote the absorption of medications, food safety, the importance of fluids and hydration, and nutrient-dense food choices. In this way, patients and clinicians can efficiently address topics of concern to most patients while preserving time in private sessions for individual evaluation and counseling.

Efficiency, however, may not be the answer to every patient's problem. Some patients may have problems when they must take HIV drugs that require refrigeration and they do not have a refrigerator. Other drugs require high-fat or low-fat meals or even no meals during dosing and need to be taken on a set schedule. If patients are homeless and have access to meals only at a soup kitchen, they have less control over meal composition or timing. Sometimes patients may not comply with follow-up appointments for medical and nutrition needs because they lack funds for transportation or day care or are simply fatigued and depressed.

Follow-up evaluation and counseling sessions can help to deter-

## FIGURE 5-2  Discharge Communication[a]

Date _____   Client _____   Record # _____   Age _____

Primary care/referring physician: _____
Risk category: 1  2  3  4   Next appt: _____
Pertinent medical history: _____
_____
_____

**General**
A&O/confused _____
_____
❑ Coping/noncoping
❑ Homebound/ bedridden
❑ Mobility with assist/s assist
❑ Self-care with assist/s assist

Vision _____
❑ Hearing
❑ Dentures
Chewing/swallowing ____
Other limitations _____
_____

**Symptoms**
❑ Diarrhea (freq/amt) _____
❑ Constipation
❑ Nausea/ vomiting
❑ Fatigue
❑ GI symptoms _____

**Self-Report of Appetite**
❑ Exc     ❑ Good
❑ Fair    ❑ Poor
Best times of day  ( ❑ am,  ❑ pm)
❑ Varies by day
Cooking facilities _____
Storage facilities _____

Who shops: _____
Who prepares: _____
Intolerance: _____
Preferences:
  Meat/sub: _____
  Dairy: _____
  Veg/fruits: _____
  Bread/grains: _____
  Fats: _____

**Physical Findings**
Height: _____    Weight: _____    Weight change: ____#/____ wk-mo    TSF: _____
                                                                                MAC: _____

Usual body weight: _____                                                   AMC: _____
Desired body weight (patient): _____
Desired body weight (RD): _____                                            % Body fat: _____

                Observation:                        Possible nutrition implications:
Nails:       _____        _____
Hair:        _____        _____
Eyes:        _____        _____
Oral/tongue: _____        _____
Skin:        _____        _____

**Laboratory Values**
TP: _____    Albumin: _____    TFN: _____    Prealb: _____    H/H: _____    CHI: _____
Na: _____    K: _____    P: _____    Cl: _____    CO$_2$: _____
Glucose: ___   Mg: _____    Ca: _____    Zn: _____    Se: _____
B-12: _____    B-6: _____    Folate: _____    Fe: _____    IBC: _____    MCV: _____
d-xylose: ___                   Schilling: ___                    Other: _____
Comment:

## FIGURE 5-2 Discharge Communication[a] (Continued)

**Problems:**  **Interventions/interactions:**  **Expected outcome:**

Knowledge:

Access:

Support:

Biochemical alteration:

DNI:

Physical exam:

Estimated energy requirements: _____   Based on: BEE x_____ IF x _____ AF _____ kcal/kg DBW/CBW

Estimated protein requirements: _____   Based on: kcal x 0.0416 _____ g protein/kg

Estimated fluid requirements: _____

Referral/ intervention recommendations:

RD signature: _____ Date sent: _____

[a]Appt indicates appointment; A&O, alert and oriented; freq/amt, frequency/amount; GI, gastrointestinal; exc, excellent; sub, substitute; veg, vegetables; TSF, triceps skinfold; MAC, midarm circumference; AMC, arm muscle circumference; RD, registered dietitian; TP, total protein; Na, sodium; K, potassium; Mg, magnesium; TFN, transferrin; P, phosporus; Ca, calcium; Schilling, Schilling test for GI absorption of vitamin B-12; prealb, prealbumin; Cl, chlorine; Zn, zinc; Fe, iron; H, hydrogen; $CO_2$, carbon dioxide; Se, selenium; IBC, iron-binding capacity; CHI, creatinine-height index; MCV, mean corpuscular volume; DNI, drug-nutrient interactions; BEE, basal energy expenditure; IF, injury factor; AF, activity factor; and DBW/CBW, desirable body weight/current body weight.

mine progress toward goals and trends in health status. Baseline and follow-up measures of fat folds, arm muscle circumference, and bioelectrical impedance measures and estimates can be recorded on flow sheets (Figure 5-5). Counseling sessions may focus on answering patient questions, completing a food intake record, managing HIV-related symptoms, and suggesting ways to improve the quality of life. More specific information on oral, enteral, and parenteral recommendations are covered in Chapters 3 and 4.

Goals in the outpatient care setting depend on the clinical status and the overall care plan goals. A patient's status may range from fully asymptomatic HIV infection to end-stage AIDS and qualification for hospice care. Therefore, goals will range from the prevention and rehabilitation of malnutrition to hospitalization and comfort care. Trends in accessing outpatient clinic services on the part of HIV-infected patients are described in a later section of this chapter (see "Use of Health Services by Persons With HIV Disease").

## Home Health Care Settings

In 1981 HIV-infected persons first learned of their diagnosis only in the last stages of the disease (6). At the time, there were no laboratory tests

## FIGURE 5.3 Sample Referral Format for Nutrition Services

Referral is made to : _____

For the following services:
- ❏ Nutrition assessment and recommendations
- ❏ Nutrition education and counseling
- ❏ Other (please specify) _____

Based on the following criteria:
- ❏ Immune dysfunction
- ❏ Recent weight loss (_____ lb over _____ wk)
- ❏ Symptoms:
  - ❏ nausea and/or vomiting
  - ❏ loss of appetite
  - ❏ lactose, fat, or other intolerance
  - ❏ mouth sores or pain on swallowing
  - ❏ difficulty chewing/swallowing
  - ❏ diarrhea
  - ❏ taste alterations
  - ❏ other _____
- ❏ Laboratory evaluation:[a]
  - ❏ decreased albumin (<32 g/L), transferrin (<2 g/dL), prealbumin (<150 mg/L)
  - ❏ decreased cholesterol (<2.6 mmol/L)
  - ❏ anemia (please specify) _____
  - ❏ Other (please specify) _____

Please return the following documentation:
- ❏ Note for chart
- ❏ Goals and monitoring plan
- ❏ Other report (please specify): _____

[a]To convert g/L albumin to g/dL, multiply g/L by 0.1. To convert g/L transferrin to mg/dL, multiply g/L by 100. To convert mg/L prealbumin to mg/dL, multiply by 0.1. To convert mmol/L cholesterol to mg/dL, multiply mmol/L by 38.7.

to confirm HIV status. Patients were hospitalized primarily in acute-care facilities and sometimes stayed there until they died. Later, as clinicians became more knowledgeable about HIV and more skilled in treating its associated infections, patients started to live longer. Before long, they were ready to be discharged from acute-care facilities. Support came in the form of community volunteers who staffed home care agencies. In 1984 a formal home care program for patients with AIDS began under the auspices of the Visiting Nurse Association and Hospice of San Francisco. One year later, the Visiting Nurse Service of New York started its own program; today, it is the world's largest home care program of its kind, serving a census of 1,800 persons with AIDS (6).

Two other factors contributing to the increased care of HIV-infected patients in the home setting include health care reform and cost containment. More hospitals are discharging patients sooner and sometimes sicker, so patients are receiving follow-up care at home. Increasing numbers of therapies such as intravenous (IV) antibiotic administration, enteral and parenteral nutrition, and even blood transfusions are conducted in home care or other outpatient settings.

Goals for nutrition intervention in home health range from basic education and prevention of malnutrition to aggressive rehabilitation

**FIGURE 5-4** Nutrition Care Standards for the Outpatient Clinic[a]

| Priority | Diagnosis | Therapy | Weight | Laboratory Data[b] | Intake | Action |
|---|---|---|---|---|---|---|
| 1 | HIV disease/AIDS, organ dysfunction, wasting syndrome, dysphagia, failure to thrive, growth failure | TPN, tube feeding | 10% weight loss/1 month, BMI <17 | BCM change, albumin <25 g/L, low prealbumin and transferrin, altered electrolytes | <60% intake for >3 d, anorexia, low intake for >7 d; special diets: renal, diabetic, low-protein | Chart review, evaluation, recommendations; coordinate nutrition services, insurance coverage, and home visit as needed; monitor monthly |
| 2 | Moderate diarrhea, active infection, chronic disease symptoms (eg, nausea) | Nephrotoxic or hepatotoxic therapy, endocrine replacement therapy, antiretrovirals, chemotherapy, hydration | >10% weight loss in 6 months, BMI <18 | Albumin <30 g/L, other values indicative of nutritional risk | <80% intake for >14d; special diets; other treatments, self-treatment; taste alterations, food aversions, other interferences with food intake | Chart review, evaluation, and recommendations; monitor quarterly |
| 3 | Hospice care | Antibiotics or other therapies with potential nutrient interactions | Short-term acute weight loss <2%/month with relative stability | | <100% intake for >1 month; special diets or diet questions | Chart review, evaluation, and recommendations; continue on request |
| 4 | Other: | | | | | |

Source: The Cutting Edge, Cary, Illinois.
[a]TPN indicates total parenteral nutrition; BMI, body mass index; and BCM, body cell mass.
[b]To convert g/L albumin to g/dL, multiply g/L by 0.1.

**FIGURE 5-5  Nutritional Monitoring Sheet**

Patient:_____   Wrist circumference:_____
Frame size:   ☐ small   ☐ medium   ☐ large

| | | | | | | | | |
|---:|---|---|---|---:|---|---|---|
| Date | | | | Date | | | |
| Weight | | | | Na | | | |
| Energy intake | | | | K | | | |
| Protein intake | | | | Ca | | | |
| BEE | | | | P | | | |
| EEE | | | | Mg | | | |
| Est protein req | | | | BUN | | | |
| Est fluid req | | | | Creatinine | | | |
| % Cal needs met | | | | Total protein | | | |
| % Pro needs met | | | | Albumin | | | |
| BIA resist/react | | | | Glucose | | | |
| BCM | | | | Cholesterol | | | |
| ECT | | | | Triglycerides | | | |
| Fat | | | | Amylase | | | |
| Phase angle | | | | Hemoglobin | | | |
| MAC | | | | Hematocrit | | | |
| Triceps SF | | | | TIBC | | | |
| Biceps SF | | | | TFN | | | |
| Subscapular SF | | | | Prealbumin | | | |
| Suprailiac SF | | | | d-xylose | | | |

BEE indicates basal energy expenditure; EEE, estimated energy expenditure; est, estimated; req, requirements; BIA, bioelectrical impedance analysis; BCM, body cell mass; ECT, extracellular tissue; MAC, midarm circumference; SF, skinfold; Na, sodium; K, potassium; Ca, calcium; P, phosphorus; Mg, magnesium; BUN, serum urea nitrogen; TIBC, total iron-binding capacity; and TFN, transferrin.

efforts. Maintenance, palliative, and hospice nutrition-related care may also be provided in a home health setting (see the section at the end of this chapter on hospice care). As in other settings, assessment should begin as early as possible. Information from the health care team members in other settings, such as the hospital dietitian, can smooth the transition to home care.

The range of home services varies between and even within agencies. Agency policy and personnel may provide the framework for the type of services provided. JCAHO nutrition care standards for home care are shown in Figure 5-6.

In the home health care setting, as in virtually every health care setting, a nurse often communicates first with the patient, even if nutrition screening or counseling is involved (7). Many dietitians in the home care field develop a basic nutrition screening tool for nurses to use with patients at home (7). In most agencies, the dietitian becomes involved when the screening indicates the need to monitor patients receiving total parenteral nutrition, to combat malnutrition, or to attend to another nutrition-related problem. Nutrition education materials, particularly handouts for the patients and families or caregivers, are the major take-home message from the dietitian. As such, these materials can commu-

**FIGURE 5.6  1997-98 Nutrition Care Standards for JCAHO[a] Accreditation for Home Care**

| | |
|---|---|
| TX.8 | Interdisciplinary nutrition care planning is performed, as appropriate |
| TX.8.1 | Authorized individuals prescribe or order nutrition therapies |
| TX.8.2 | Responsibilities for preparing, storing, distributing, and administering nutrition therapy are defined and assigned |
| TX.8.3 | Each patient's nutrition therapy is distributed in a safe, accurate, and timely manner |
| TX.8.4 | Each patient's nutrition therapy is administered in a safe, accurate, and timely manner |
| TX.8.5 | Each patient's nutrition status is monitored on an ongoing basis |
| TX.8.6 | The organization provides appropriate nutrition therapy when diets or diet schedules are altered |

Source: *Comprehensive Accreditation Manual for Home Care, 1997-98.* Oakbrook Terrace, Ill: Joint Commission on Accreditation of Healthcare Organizations; 1996:201-205. Reprinted with permission.

[a]JCAHO Joint Commission on Accreditation of Healthcare Organizations.

nicate important information about food safety and ways to relieve gastrointestinal (GI) symptoms, among other topics.

Many home care agencies are developing clinical pathways and other procedures for carrying out medical nutrition therapy (7). This is also an important part of program development for disease management with which the dietitian can be involved.

Carefully delineated referral criteria and standards of care will dictate the access to dietitian services to assess, recommend, and implement nutrition care. As in the acute-care setting, nutrition support teams can be formed in home health settings. The support of the physician and the involvement of the dietitian, pharmacist, nurse, social worker, physical therapist, and other personnel as appropriate are essential to the successful integration of nutrition therapies.

## PREPARATION FOR EMPLOYMENT IN HOME HEALTH

As patients live longer and budgetary cutbacks in traditional health care settings increase, more dietitians specializing in HIV may be needed as employees or consultants to home care agencies. Dietitians who want to enter the home health field should obtain experience in critical care and community nutrition (7). Experience in a clinical setting prepares the dietitian to conduct nutrition screening, assessment, and counseling. Community experience allows the dietitian to identify and tap into community resources. Additionally, dietitians may find it helpful to have multilingual skills.

It is also recommended that dietitians seeking jobs caring for patients with HIV disease volunteer at a nonprofit agency and attend conferences on HIV, AIDS, and nutrition (Marcy Fenton, MS, RD, personal communication, January 2, 1997). Expertise in nutrition support is a qualification that the American Society for Parenteral and Enteral Nutrition (ASPEN) regards as important for a dietitian to have as a member of the home health care team (8). A survey of dietitians in home care found that important skills were counseling patients, conducting dietary histories, providing education to caregivers, and developing a care plan (9).

## Use of Health Services by Persons With HIV Disease

The severity of HIV disease does not always predict which health service patients and their providers will select or how long they will use the service. In one urban multicenter study, when patients' CD4 lymphocyte counts decreased from a range of 200 to 500/mm$^3$ to less than 50/mm$^3$ the number of inpatient days over the total period from diagnosis to death quadrupled (10). But a low CD4 cell count did not necessarily predict longer hospitalization, especially over time. The number of inpatient days among those with a CD4 cell count of 50/mm$^3$ or less was cut almost in half from 24 days in 1988 to 12.5 days in 1990 (11).

Race can affect how often a particular health service is used. In the same study it was found that whites visited HIV clinics more frequently than did people of color, and this difference grew when the CD4 cell counts decreased to their lowest level (<50/mm$^3$). People of color had more hospital admissions. This finding is supported by results from other studies showing that the use of preventive health care measures and the visitation of emergency rooms may vary according to race (11, 12).

Another study, the Multicenter AIDS Cohort Study (MACS), published results of the impact of immunosuppression on the use of three different types of health care services: hospitalization, outpatient visits to a physician's office or hospital-based clinic, and the emergency room (13). Participating in the study were 3,447 homosexual or bisexual men in different stages of HIV infection. Low-income patients used emergency rooms more than their counterparts with private health insurance. The researchers commented that the emergency room was an expensive way to deliver primary care, especially since its use was not associated with a low CD4 cell count. Furthermore, this trend reflects a gap in the continuum of care for patients with public health insurance or those who are uninsured. In this study, Medicaid was used more frequently as HIV disease progressed, and emergency room admissions of Medicaid patients were higher than those of patients with private insurance. Race did not predict which services patients used. Deteriorating immunologic status was not associated with longer hospitalizations. Still, according to MACS, hospitalization of patients with AIDS tended to last twice as long as the average hospitalization, although the patients enrolled in MACS had shorter hospitalizations on average than did other populations of patients with AIDS (13).

Cost is another factor that can differentiate one health care delivery system from another. God's Love We Deliver (GLWD), a nonprofit agency for homebound persons with HIV in New York City, compared costs of its home-delivered meals to hospitalization for malnutrition related to HIV disease (14). The agency estimated that if its meals are able to prevent malnutrition-associated hospitalization for a total of $13 a day per client, cost savings could average $1,100 per day. This underscores the potential value of preventive nutrition care.

Even though community-based nutrition services can lower the cost of health care by potentially reducing the number of hospitalizations (15) and supporting recuperation from opportunistic infections

(16), nutrition services in the community may not be used as fully as expected by persons with HIV infection (17). In a needs assessment survey, GLWD (14) found that many clients who were eligible for free food and food stamps were not using these services. A study in Ohio concurred about the underutilization of nutrition services (17). Of the 22 survey participants, all of whom had HIV infection or AIDS, 14 believed that they could benefit from seeing a nutritionist or dietitian as part of their home health care package, but only one person had received any nutrition intervention. Inadequate health insurance and lack of funding from the state Medicaid program for nutrition services seemed to account for the unmet nutrition needs in this study. To prevent this situation from occurring in their states, dietitians in Oregon, Hawaii, Tennessee, Minnesota, Vermont, New Hampshire, Montana, and other states have worked to obtain coverage for their services in their state Medicaid Programs (18).

Access to health care services for HIV-infected persons is an important issue. Public health workers are reaching out to low-income persons with HIV and AIDS who are medically underserved, for example, women, children, adolescents, minorities, and substance abusers. Outreach efforts include primary care services in medicine, nutrition, dentistry, and mental health through the HIV Early Intervention Services Programs (19). Funded by the Ryan White Comprehensive AIDS Resources Emergency Act, these programs are available to agencies such as community migrant health centers, outpatient clinics, public health departments, family planning organizations, gay and lesbian organizations, health care programs for the homeless, and comprehensive hemophilia centers. Many of these agencies employ full-time or part-time dietitians. Teams evaluate HIV Early Intervention Services Programs around the country, according to team leader Laura McNally Kruse, MPH, RD, a project officer and nutrition consultant with the Bureau of Primary Health Care (personal communication, December 1996). Programs include a lottery for protease inhibitors in Texas, where 500 people with AIDS are clamoring to receive these new drugs.

## Managed Care

Because managed care is a relatively new concept compared with the traditional health care system, its role in serving patients with HIV has yet to be elucidated in the literature. What is well established is that managed care is a payment method in the health care system that focuses its attention on using health care resources effectively and cost-efficiently (20). Unlike a fee-for-service system, some managed care organizations try to curtail the spiraling costs of health care in the United States by emphasizing ambulatory care, reducing the length of inpatient treatment, and promoting the continuum of care in the community. Established first in the private sector, managed care attempts to accomplish these goals by stipulating conditions for participation, reducing reliance on higher priced specialists, requiring prior approval for non-emergency hospital services, and refusing to pay for treatment deemed wasteful (20).

In the United States, the number of persons enrolled in managed care programs continues to increase as the private and public sectors strive for new ways to cut costs of insuring health care for their employees. Critics of this system state that patients who need to see a specialist may find they have restricted access because of more stringent criteria or financial incentives. However, the type and quality of health care insurance varies from one state to the next and from one agency to another.

A large provider of managed care in southern California, Med Partners/Friendly Hills Health Care Network, has seven registered dietitians on staff who see 50 to 60 patients a month (Ellyn Silverman, MPH, RD, personal communication, December 8, 1996). All newly diagnosed HIV-positive patients are referred to a registered dietitian, who performs a baseline nutrition assessment. Within this managed care organization, nutrition care is a covered benefit of various health plans and is free to plan members. A task force with various health professionals, including a dietitian, developed medical and nutrition care protocols for HIV-infected patients within the network. Also developed was a curriculum aimed at preventing HIV infection. This managed care plan has contracts with health maintenance organizations where dietitians provide continuing medical education on HIV to health care personnel. When patients enrolled in this plan receive a diagnosis, they are sent to a dietitian as part of the treatment plan. Another source of referrals includes hospitals that have contracts with managed care organizations to refer patients who need follow-up once they leave the hospital. In turn, these patients may be referred to a community-based nutrition service. Patients receive initial nutrition assessments through this managed care plan, as well as subsequent nutrition counseling services as needed. Some common problems encountered include side effects from medications or vitamin megadosing, diarrhea, loss of appetite, poor sanitation practices at home, and water-borne and food-borne illnesses.

Managed care is a trend that is expected to grow. Dietitians who can document to managed care organizations the cost savings of their services have reason to be optimistic that expanding professional opportunities await them. In addition, educating health care providers on nutritional outcomes data is key to obtaining referrals in this new system.

## Community-Based Nutrition Programs in AIDS Care
### BASIC SERVICES

To help the patient with HIV disease make the transition from hospital to home, the clinician needs to know which food and nutrition resources are available in the community. Community-based nutrition support consists of a variety of tangible and intangible assistance to protect the nutritional health of patients through private and public funding. On any given day, clinicians could find that the following services are readily available in a major metropolitan area and frequently in a rural community as well:

- Ready-to-eat or frozen meals delivered to the client's home (14). In the past decade, home-delivered meals have been established

in almost 20 major cities in the United States to meet the nutrition needs of homebound persons with AIDS (15) (see Appendix D).
- Congregate meals. These are meals prepared by either an agency or a group of clients at one of their homes or at an agency site. (14)
- Food pantries. Groceries are delivered to the client's home or picked up in a central location by the client (14).
- Food stamps. The US Department of Agriculture (USDA) provides food stamps in the form of grocery store coupons to welfare offices or state social service agencies to distribute to needy recipients.
- The Special Supplemental Food Program for Women, Infants, and Children (WIC). Also administered by the USDA, WIC provides healthy foods and nutrition education to low-income women who are pregnant or breast-feeding and to their young children.
- Nutrition education. New York-based GLWD conducts workshops for clients on issues such as ways to save money on groceries, food safety, and dietary strategies to ease stomach problems for HIV-related illnesses (14). Four full-time HIV nutrition specialists are on staff at this agency to meet client needs. Education materials that are culturally appropriate are available on nutrition and HIV disease (16). At AIDS Project Los Angeles (APLA), California's largest AIDS service organization and one of the largest agencies of its type in the country, one to two nutrition presentations are held weekly, in addition to a monthly forum on nutrition and HIV featuring three dietitians (Marcy Fenton, MS, RD, personal communication, January 2, 1997). A variety of subjects are presented, such as ways to increase body cell mass, management of diarrhea, food and water safety, and nausea reduction.
- Nutrition counseling. Many community agencies provide counseling to patients (15). At APLA, 20 to 50 clients are seen each month, in addition to an equal number of telephone consultations. God's Love We Deliver also provides nutrition counseling by telephone to clients classified as "high priority" (16).

## COMMUNITY-BASED NUTRITION STANDARDS

Community-based nutrition standards of care include those issued by GLWD and at Food and Friends, an agency based in Washington, DC. Examples of these standards include the following (14; Barbara Blesi, RD, Food and Friends, personal communication, December 7, 1996):

- The daily nutrition intake of HIV-infected persons is set at a minimum of 2,400 kcal by GLWD. The standard of Food and Friends is also set at 2,400 kcal, derived by calculating the average weight of 25% of its clients (148 lb) and then providing 35 kcal/kg of body weight.
- Fat accounts for 30% to 35% of kilocalories of food served by GLWD, but the proportion of fat can be increased to 40% to provide for extra energy or to include comfort foods.

- The protein standard of GLWD allots 90 to 105 g (based on 1.5 to 2 g of protein per kilogram of body weight to promote weight gain). Similarly, Food and Friends has set a protein level of 1.5 to 2 g/kg of body weight for each client. In the event of chronic diarrhea or hypermetabolism, GLWD increases the protein level to 2 to 2.5 g (14).
- At least 100% of the RDA for vitamins and minerals should be met in the 2,400-kcal menu. God's Love We Deliver suggests that clients see their physicians for recommendations for receiving nutrient supplementation. Because more HIV-infected women than previously are availing themselves of the services at Food and Friends, calcium and iron needs may increase. Three years ago women constituted under 10% of the agency's clientele. In 1996, that figure rose to approximately 25%.
- Commercial nutritional supplements are provided to the clients by GLWD.
- Regarding fluids, GLWD recommends 30 mL/kg of body weight for adults and 35 mL/kg of weight for children. Food and Friends recommends eight to 10 glasses of water a day.

Community nutrition agencies frequently receive requests for vegetarian meals and therapeutic diets such as renal and diabetic diets (Barbara Blesi, RD, personal communication, December 7, 1996). God's Love We Deliver provides a modified diet for renal patients and offers smaller portions of food as well as special protein-rich foods because of vegetarian preferences or allergies (14). Therapeutic considerations for this clientele include foods modified in acid, fiber, and dairy content (see Table 5-1) (15). Other diseases aside from AIDS-associated illnesses may necessitate diabetic, renal, and hepatic diets.

## NUTRITION CARE AND MORE

Most nutrition agencies serving the needs of HIV-infected persons began as a response to inadequate resources for food leading to the risk of starvation-style malnutrition (14). Today the goal of most is to intervene as soon as HIV infection is diagnosed, to prevent weight loss, preserve muscle mass, and avoid food-borne illnesses. This requires nutrient- and protein-dense meals and snacks that are both safe and appetizing.

Because patients with HIV are prone to GI ailments, many community agencies educate their staff, volunteers, and clients about food safety (14). Project Open Hand in San Francisco addresses the issue of food safety by providing clients with printed guidelines, plus regular tips in a monthly newsletter, and by delivering hot foods to an alternate site if the client is not at home. Two other agencies, the Chicken Brigade in Seattle and Open Hand in Atlanta, also educate their clients about food safety in addition to equipping them with microwave ovens (donated by supporters) for reheating food safely (14).

As noted earlier, many agencies provide groceries for clients with HIV disease. Food and Friends has a service called Groceries-To-Go, which includes stable, easy-to-prepare foods plus five frozen entrees. The groceries are delivered once a week to clients who live many miles away from Food and Friends (Barbara Blesi, RD, personal communication, December 7, 1996). At APLA's food pantry, $2 million worth of groceries a year are distributed to 1,600 needy clients (Marcy Fenton, MS, RD, personal communication, January 2, 1997).

Substance abuse is just one problem that public health dietitians specializing in the care of HIV-infected clients may encounter. Many of these clients are poor or homeless and may be unable to maintain strict standards of hygiene. Dietitians need to be flexible and nonjudgmental, since they serve clients who may come from different cultures (12). Also, because people with AIDS are now living longer, HIV specialists must deal with a whole new set of issues: those facing the chronically ill (Laura Kruse, personal communication, December 1996). Despite the depressing side of this disease, those who work on behalf of people with AIDS have a high level of commitment and dedication (Laura Kruse, personal communication, December 1996), and dietitians who work in this field can know that they play an important role.

## Hospice Setting

Hospice care emphasizes a philosophy of treatment during the final stages of life. The National Hospice Organization states that "hospice affirms life . . . neither hastens nor postpones death [and] recognizes dying as a normal process whether or not resulting from disease." (23) The goals of hospice are to relieve pain and other symptoms and allow the patient to live in comfort and with dignity during the final months, weeks, or days of life.

The hospice philosophy integrates a team approach to address the physical, psychosocial, and spiritual needs of the patient. Nutritional rehabilitation becomes a lower priority, and universal assessment of nutritional status becomes a question of the benefit vs burden of the process to the patient. Figure 5-7 shows JCAHO guidelines for nutrition services in the hospice setting.

Screening and assessment criteria are aimed at maximizing quality time with family and friends. Information gathered from medical records and health care providers may include chief complaints, medical goals, prognosis, level of pain, cultural background, and level of function. Complete panels of biochemical indexes, invasive testing procedures, and in some cases even body weight may not be appropriate. Drug-nutrient interactions and records of dietary intake play an important role in assessment, as these factors may affect patient comfort and interaction with loved ones. The patient's ability and desire to eat, as

---

**FIGURE 5.7 Nutrition Care Standards for JCAHO[a] Accreditation for Facility-Based Hospice Care**

TX.9.  Menus are planned and posted in areas accessible to hospice patients
TX.10. Responsibilities for preparing and distributing food and nutrition products are fulfilled

Source: *Comprehensive Accreditation Manual for Home Care, 1997-98.* Oakbrook Terrace, Ill: Joint Commission on Accreditation of Healthcare Organizations; 1996:205. Reprinted with permission.

[a]JCAHO Joint Commission on Accreditation of Healthcare Organizations.

well as the patient's and family's perception of eating, are also pertinent to nutrition care planning.

Hospice care may be provided in the patient's residence or a loved one's home, group residence, hospital, skilled nursing facility, or other sites. A goal of therapy in the acute-care setting may be to stabilize the patient enough for discharge into settings more conducive to implementing full hospice care. In an institutional setting, food service and food safety become important issues to address.

Hospice care for HIV disease may differ somewhat from traditional hospice programs. It may be difficult to establish a timed prognosis for patients with HIV disease. Guidelines and admission criteria may differ because of the patient's desires for aggressive treatment or preventive therapies for some complications and palliative care for other conditions. For instance, IV ganciclovir, administered to prevent blindness caused by cytomegalovirus-associated retinitis, may be a quality-of-life issue during the final stages of HIV disease. The use of hydration and nutrition support in terminally ill patients has stirred controversy over guidelines on the purpose and use of this type of therapy (24).

## HIV/AIDS Medical Nutrition Therapy Protocol

The HIV/AIDS Medical Nutrition Therapy (MNT) protocol (21) is a template that can be used in many health care settings (see Appendix B). It was developed to help dietitians communicate the benefits of medical nutrition therapy to other health care professionals and managed care organizations. There are three major outcomes to assess: clinical, functional, and behavioral (21).

### CLINICAL OUTCOMES

Clinical outcomes for patients with HIV infection or AIDS measure biochemical indexes, anthropometric data, and clinical signs and symptoms. Among the expected outcomes in the clinical category are to minimize weight loss; prevent dehydration; keep laboratory values from declining during early and symptomatic stages of the HIV infection; and treat diarrhea, nausea, vomiting, and dysphagia.

### FUNCTIONAL OUTCOMES

Functional outcomes measure how well the patient is able to carry out the activities of daily living, or ADL (see level 2 nutrition screening in Chapter 2). The ADL needs to be assessed in the inpatient setting before the patient is discharged in case assisted care is needed at home. Every few months, the outpatient or home health dietitian needs to reassess the patient's ADL in the event that economic conditions deteriorate, drug abuse occurs, or the patient's medical condition warrants additional care.

### BEHAVIORAL OUTCOMES

Behavioral outcomes assess the changes in the patient's actions for following safe and beneficial nutrition and dietary practices recommended by the dietitian. Can the patient verbalize food and water sanitation practices to follow at home and state why they are important? How does the patient plan to maintain weight once he or she is released from the hospital? Does the patient know which foods are appropriate when extra energy is needed? Can the patient cook? If not, does the dietitian know how to arrange for meal delivery if needed? (See Appendix D for a listing of nutrition-based services in the community.)

When patients with HIV disease suffer from debilitating fatigue, being shunted through the health system is a demanding job. Providing the same medical history repeatedly to five or even 10 health care professionals in a month is not unusual. To prevent frustration and save time, while concurrently allowing the patient to rest and recover, the dietitian can obtain specifics about each case from the referral source. The length of the nutrition assessment session will vary according to the patient's needs and strength (22).

## Summary

Although there are many standard nutrition screening and assessment criteria, the information available and its application to nutrition care plans for patients with HIV disease vary according to the health care setting. The category of disease, patient status, appropriate health care goals, attitudes and practices of patients, access to health care, and economics of the health care system all determine the types of assessment and intervention available within each setting. New drugs and the commitment of dedicated health care workers in the field offer hope. However, the indigence and suffering of many patients and the fear and frustrations of some dietitians and their colleagues can cloud the picture. The challenge for the dietitian specializing in HIV disease is to overcome barriers and find a balance in providing the best care possible in every health care setting.

*References*

1. Position of The American Dietetic Association and The Canadian Dietetic Association. Nutrition intervention in the care of persons with human immunodeficiency virus infection. *J Am Diet Assoc.* 1994; 1042-1045.
2. Whitney EN, Cataldo CB, Rolfes SR. The team approach. In: *Understanding Normal and Clinical Nutrition.* St Paul, Minn: West Publishing; 1994:589-591.
3. Flanel DF, Fairchild MM. Continuous quality improvement in inpatient clinical nutrition services. *J Am Diet Assoc.* 1995;95:65-74.
4. Krasker GD, Balogun LB. 1995 JCAHO standards: development and relevance to dietetics practice. *J Am Diet Assoc.* 1995;95:240-243.
5. Beaudette T, ed. *Seminars in Nutrition: Nutritional Aspects of AIDS and HIV Infection.* 1995;14:1-17.
6. Ungvarski PJ. Challenges for the urban home health care provider. *Nurs Clin North Am.* 1996;31:81-95.
7. Hahn NI. Home is where the jobs are. *J Am Diet Assoc.* 1996;96:332.
8. American Society for Parenteral and Enteral Nutrition. Standards for home nutrition support. *Nutr Clin Pract.* 1992;7:65-69.
9. Arensberg MBF, Schiller R. Dietitians in home care: a survey of current practice. *J Am Diet Assoc.* 1996;96:347-353.

10. Piette JD, Mor V, Mayer K, Zierler S, Wachtel T. The effects of immune status and race on health service use among people with HIV disease. *Am J Public Health.* 1993;83:510-514.
11. Piette J, Stein M, Mor V, et al. Patterns of secondary prophylaxis with aerosol pentamidine among persons with AIDS. *J AIDS.* 1991;4:826-828.
12. Mor V, Fleischman JA, Dresser M, Piette J. Variation in health service use among HIV infected patients. *Med Care.* 1992;30:17-29.
13. Zucconi SL, Jacobson LP, Schrager LK, Kass NE, Lave JR, Carson CA, Morgenstern H, Arno PS, Graham NM. Impact of immunosuppression on health care use by men in the Multicenter AIDS Cohort Study (MACS). *J AIDS.* 1994;7:607-616.
14. Abdale F. *Community-Based Nutrition Support for People Living With HIV and AIDS: A Technical Assistance Manual.* New York, NY: God's Love We Deliver; 1995.
15. Kraak VI. Home-delivered meal programs for homebound people with HIV/AIDS. *J Am Diet Assoc.* 1995;95:476-481.
16. Kaplan CR: Community-based nutrition support: home-delivered meals reach people living with AIDS. *Networking News.* Spring 1996; 8:5, 11.
17. Udine LM, Rothkopf MM. Utilization of home health care services and HIV infection: a pilot study in Ohio. *J Am Diet Assoc.* 1994;94:83-85.
18. State and federal efforts to trim health care costs embrace Medicaid waivers and managed care. Legislative Highlights. *J Am Diet Assoc.* 1995;95:750.
19. *Health Care and HIV: Nutritional Guide for Providers and Clients.* Vienna, Va: Bureau of Primary Health Care, US Department of Health and Human Resources; 1996.
20. Edelman RD, Johnson RK, Coulston AM. Securing the inclusion of medical nutrition therapy in managed care health systems. *J Am Diet Assoc.* 1995;95:1100-1102.
21. HIV/AIDS medical nutrition therapy protocol. In: *Medical Nutrition Therapy Across the Continuum of Care.* Chicago, Ill: The American Dietetic Association, 1996.
22. Licavoli L, Hahn NI. Dietetics goes into therapy. *J Am Diet Assoc.* 1995;95:751-752.
23. Hastings Center. *Guidelines on the Termination of Life-sustaining Treatment and the Care of the Dying.* Bloomington, Ind: Indiana University Press; 1997.
24. Edelstein S, Anderson S. Bioethics and dietetics: education and attitudes. *J Am Diet Assoc.* 1991;91:546-548.

# Appendix A
# Glossary of HIV and AIDS Terms

**acquired immunodeficiency syndrome (AIDS)**—A secondary immunodeficiency disease that results from infection by HIV. It is characterized by a diverse spectrum of disorders, including opportunistic infections, malignancies, neurologic dysfunctions, wasting, and gastrointestinal ailments.

**acute retroviral syndrome (ARS)**—The first condition in primary HIV infection. It causes flulike symptoms.

**AIDS**—See acquired immunodeficiency syndrome.

**AIDS-related complex (ARC)**—Term previously used to describe a level of symptoms experienced by persons infected with HIV who did not qualify for a diagnosis of AIDS.

**alternative therapy**—An alternative to conventional medicine, sometimes termed holistic or complementary therapy, or integrative medicine. A wide range of therapies is grouped under this heading, including biofeedback, osteopathy, acupuncture, chiropractic treatment, homeopathy, herbal treatments, naturopathy, and nutrition.

**antibody**—An immunoglobulin molecule formed in response to invading foreign material. Antibodies usually confer protection against targeted substances to develop immunity, but this process does not occur with the formation of HIV antibodies. This is the substance that is tested for in HIV testing.

**antigen**—A foreign substance that enters the body and induces a specific immune response by forming an antibody.

**ARC**—See AIDS-related complex.

**ARS**—See acute retroviral syndrome.

**blood-borne disease**—An infectious disease involving agents that are carried in the bloodstream (eg, HIV and hepatitis B).

**candidiasis**—A fungal infection that may occur as an opportunistic infection in the mouth or throat (thrush), esophagus, vagina, or skin. Other sites may be involved less frequently.

**CDC**—See Centers for Disease Control and Prevention.

**CD4**—A molecule on the T-helper cells, macrophages, and some other cells to which HIV binds itself.

**cell-mediated immunity**—The immune response carried out by helper and killer T cells. Helper T cells orchestrate the immune system's defense, and killer T cells destroy infected cells.

**Centers for Disease Control and Prevention (CDC)**—Federal agency in the US Department of Health and Human Services that provides health and safety guidelines and statistical monitoring data.

**CMV**—See cytomegalovirus.

**cofactor**—Something that increases the likelihood of developing a disease (eg, malnutrition or stress).

*Cryptosporidium*—A genus of protozoan parasites that cause severe intestinal wall damage and protracted diarrhea, which may lead to severe dehydration and malnutrition.

**cytokine**—A hormonelike protein that is released by certain cells to regulate immune cell activity; for example, T cells use cytokine modulators.

**cytomegalovirus (CMV)**—A viral infection that may cause loss of organ function where the infection is found (eg, loss of sight if the eye is infected).

**disinfectant**—A chemical used to destroy disease agents (eg, bleach).

**ELISA**—See enzyme-linked immunosorbent assay.

**enzyme-linked immunosorbent assay (ELISA)**—A blood test used to detect HIV antibodies. Results are confirmed by a Western blot test.

**FDA**—See Food and Drug Administration.

**Food and Drug Administration (FDA)**—The federal government agency that regulates the testing and approval of new drugs before their marketing.

**fungus**—Microscopic organism classification, which includes yeast and molds.

**gp120**—Glycoprotein 120. A glycosylated (sugar-containing) protein, gp120 is attached to the HIV envelope (outer covering or "coat") used to attach to CD4 binding sites on targeted cells. It is attached to the envelope by another glycoprotein (gp41).

**hemophilia**—An inherited blood disorder of impaired clotting.

**hepatitis B**—A viral infection that affects the liver. It is transmitted through blood and sexual contact.

**herpes simplex**—A virus that causes acute disease characterized by groups of watery blisters on the skin and mucous membranes of the lips, genitals, or anus. Type 1 mainly affects the lips; type 2 mainly affects the genitals.

**HIV**—See human immunodeficiency virus.

**HIV disease**—Term used to describe the spectrum of HIV infection, including asymptomatic and symptomatic stages.

**hospice**—A program offering compassionate care in the home or institutional setting for terminally ill people.

**HTLV-III**—See human T-cell lymphotropic virus, type III.

**human immunodeficiency virus (HIV)**—The virus that causes AIDS. HIV-1 is found in the United States, whereas HIV-2 is found primarily in Africa.

**human T-cell lymphotropic virus, type III (HTLV-III)**—The early term for HIV-1.

**immunoglobulin**—A class of antibodies that protect against disease. Intravenous administration of immunoglobulin G (IgG) is common in children and some adults with HIV disease.

**incidence**—The rate or number of new cases of a disease or condition over a time period.

**incubation**—The time from infection to the onset of symptoms of an infectious disease.

**infection**—An invasion of the body by disease agent (viral, fungal, bacterial).

**infectious disease**—A disease caused by or transmitted by a biologic agent. Diseases differ in their infectiousness and contagiousness (transmission); for example, HIV is highly infectious (disease causing) but is not transmitted easily or casually (through ordinary social contact).

**interferons**—Cytokines produced by the immune system that inhibit viral infection.

**interleukin-2**—Cytokine produced by the immune system that stimulates T cells and some B cells to proliferate. It was formerly called T-cell growth factor.

**Kaposi's sarcoma**—A cancer that may involve skin, mucous membrane, and lymph nodes. It may appear as purplish or red spots and is usually seen in immunodeficient states.

**LAV**—See lymphadenopathy-associated virus.

**lentivirus**—A type of retroviruses found in sheep, horses, and goats. The human immunodeficiency virus is a member of this subfamily. Lentivirus means "slow virus."

**lesion**—Abnormal change in the tissue or structure of an organ or body part due to injury or disease. An example is a sore.

**lymphadenopathy-associated virus (LAV)**—The early name for HIV-1.

**lymph glands**—Glands located in the groin, neck, armpits, and other parts of the body which contain lymphocytes.

**lymphocytes**—White blood cells essential to immune function. Examples are T cells and B cells.

**lymphoma**—Cancer of lymphoid tissue. Hodgkin's and non-Hodgkin's lymphoma are included in HIV disease.

**macrophage**—A type of white cell that devours invading organisms. It is used by HIV as a vehicle to travel to distant sites and infect new cells.

**MAI/MAC**—See *Mycobacterium avium-intracellulare/M avium* complex.

**Medicaid**—The federal and state health insurance program that pays certain medical expenses for people whose income falls below the poverty level, as set by each state.

**Medicare**—The federal health insurance program that pays certain medical expenses for people who are disabled, are 65 years of age or older, or have chronic kidney disease.

**meningitis**—Infection and inflammation of the membranes that cover the brain and spinal cord.

**monocyte**—A young macrophage.

**mucous membrane**—The lining or membrane of body passages that have an outside opening. Glands in the membrane produce mucus. Examples are the lining of the mouth and the vagina.

***Mycobacterium avium-intracellulare/M avium* complex (MAI/MAC)**—A bacterial infection that can affect most internal organs. It is associated with enlarged lymph nodes, weight loss, and diarrhea.

**National Institute of Allergy and Infectious Diseases (NIAID)**—A part of the National Institutes of Health.

**National Institutes of Health (NIH)**—The federal agency of the US Public Health Service. The NIH's 13 institutes support and conduct research, train scientists and doctors, and publish scientific reports.

**neutropenia**—An abnormally low number of neutrophils, white cells that defend against fungus and bacteria.

**NIAID**—See National Institute of Allergy and Infectious Diseases.

**NIH**—See National Institutes of Health.

**opportunistic infection**—One of various infections that occur in immune deficiency. An example is *Pneumocystis carinii* pneumonia.

**orphan drug**—Drugs developed for rare diseases.

**p24 antigen**—A measure of free viral antigen. It is a marker for viral load.

**PCP**—See *Pneumocystis carinii* pneumonia.

**PCR**—See polymerase chain reaction.

**perinatal transmission**—Transmission of an infection to an infant before or during birth.

**persistent generalized lymphadenopathy (PGL)**—It is marked by swollen lymph glands without an apparent cause and is seen in HIV-positive persons.

**PGL**—See persistent generalized lymphadenopathy.

**phase I trials**—Clinical trials which involve small numbers of healthy volunteers to determine a drug's safety.

**phase II trials**—Clinical trials involving a small number of subjects with the condition being investigated, to evaluate the safety and effectiveness of the targeted drug.

**phase III trials**—Clinical trials involving a large number of patients with the disease being investigated, to verify a drug's long-term effectiveness and safety, compared with no treatment or other treatments.

*Pneumocystis carinii* **pneumonia (PCP)**—Pneumonia caused by a parasite that poses a threat only to immune-compromised persons.

**polymerase chain reaction (PCR)**—A test that detects HIV by its genetic material, even in minute amounts or hidden in a white blood cell.

**prevalence**—The total number of cases of a disease in a population over a time period.

**prophylaxis**—Preventive treatment to preserve health and prevent the spread of disease.

**prospective cohort**—In an epidemiological study, a group of individuals with a similar characteristic who are observed over a time period. An example is a cohort of persons with a risk factor compared with those who do not have a risk factor.

**prospective study**—A trial that follows events from beginning to end over a time period.

**protease inhibitor**—A new class of medications aimed at HIV protease to prevent HIV maturation. Protease inhibitors include saquinavir mesylate, ritonavir, indinavir sulfate, and nelfinavir mesylate. These medications have moderate to severe side effect during the first weeks of therapy. However, combined with other drugs, protease inhibitors are improving the survival rates of HIV-infected persons.

**provirus**—The precursor of a virus that is integrated into the DNA of the infected cell waiting for a stimulus to produce complete copies of the original virus.

**respite care**—Short-term care of chronically ill people provided to give their caregivers a break.

**retrovirus**—A type of virus that passes genetic information to the infected cell "in reverse" or by transcribing its RNA (as opposed to DNA) with the enzyme reverse transcriptase to DNA to incorporate into the cell's genetic machinery. HIV is a retrovirus.

**reverse transcriptase**—An enzyme produced by retroviruses, which enables them to produce DNA from their original RNA.

**risk behavior**—An activity that puts a person at risk for disease.

**risk group**—A statistical description of people thought to share a common feature that puts them at increased risk for contracting a disease.

**safer sex**—Sexual practices that do not involve the exchange of blood, semen, or vaginal fluid.

**sensitivity**—The likelihood that a response will be seen to even small amounts of infection.

**seroconversion**—A change from the apparent absence of antibodies to the presence of antibodies in the blood for an infectious agent.

**seropositive**—The tested presence of particular antibodies in the serum.

**shingles**—Inflammation of nerve endings brought about by the same virus that causes chicken pox. Shingles is an opportunistic infection in immune deficiency.

**specificity**—The likelihood that a response will not be seen when no infection exists.

**tat**—Transactivator of transcription. This regulatory gene is responsible for the burst of viral replication in HIV-infected T cells. Other such genes are the gag (group-specific antigen), pol (polymerase), env (envelope), rev (regulator of virion protein expression), vif (virion infectivity factor), vpu (virion productivity factor u), and nef (negative regulatory factor); together they regulate viral growth and the relationship to its host cell.

**TB**—See tuberculosis.

**T cell**—White blood cell that regulates the immune system and controls B-cell and macrophage functions. It includes the T lymphocyte and the T-helper cell.

**toxoplasmosis**—A disease resulting from infection with the protozoa *Toxoplasma gondii*. It may involve the heart, lungs, adrenal glands, pancreas, and testes; frequently it causes encephalitis, an inflammation of the brain.

**tuberculosis (TB)**—A contagious disease that primarily affects the lungs. It is common in HIV.

**vaccine**—A substance made from modified or denatured viruses or bacteria, used to confer immunity and protect people against a particular disease.

**vector**—A living host that carries disease agents from an infected host to an uninfected host.

**vertical transmission**—Transmission of HIV from mother to child during pregnancy, childbirth, or breast-feeding.

**viral load**—The amount of virus in the body expressed in copies per milliliter. It is used to measure the degree of illness.

**virus**—A minute infectious agent that requires a host cell to survive and often destroys the host cell. Most viruses inject DNA into the host cell to take over reproductive function. HIV is a retrovirus that injects RNA into the host cell (see "retrovirus").

**wasting syndrome**—Extreme weight loss, diarrhea, weakness, and fever. It is an AIDS-defining illness.

**Western blot**—A blood test to detect antibodies to HIV. It is used to confirm ELISA.

**white blood cell**—A blood cell with the primary function of fighting infection. It includes T cells, B cells, macrophages, and monocytes.

# Appendix B
# Nutrition Assessment

# B-1 HIV/AIDS Medical Nutrition Therapy Protocol

## HIV/AIDS
### Medical Nutrition Therapy Protocol
**Setting: Ambulatory Care** (Adult 18+ years old)

**Number of sessions:** see level of care for number of sessions

| No. of interventions | Length of contact | Time between interventions | Cost/charge |
|---|---|---|---|
| Level of care 1 F/U at least 2/year | 60 minutes initial 15-30 minutes F/U session | based on assessment and/or need | |
| Level of care 2 F/U at least 2-6/year | 30-60 minutes initial 15-30 minutes F/U session | based on assessment and/or need | |
| Level of care 3 & 4 F/U as needed | 30-60 minutes initial 15-30 minutes F/U session | based on assessment and/or need | |

### Expected Outcomes of Medical Nutrition Therapy

| Outcome assessment factors | Baseline Intervention 1 | Eval of Intervention 2 | Eval of Intervention 3 | Expected outcome | Ideal/goal value |
|---|---|---|---|---|---|
| **Clinical Outcomes** | | | | | |
| • Biochemical parameters (measure <15 days prior to nutrition session) | | | | During stage I and II stay within normal levels Lab values to stabilize | Albumin 3.5-5.0 mg/dL Prealbumin 19-43 mg/dL HgB > 12 g/dL (F) > 14 g/dL (M) Hct > 38% (F) > 44% (M) Cholesterol 100-200 mg/dL Triglycerides < 500 mg/dL |
| Albumin, prealbumin | ✓ | ✓ | ✓ | | |
| CBC | ✓ | ✓ | ✓ | | |
| Cholesterol, triglycerides | ✓ | ✓ | ✓ | | |
| CD4, CD8, viral load | ✓ | ✓ | ✓ | | |
| BUN, creatinine | ✓ | ✓ | ✓ | | |
| Vitamins/minerals | ✓ | ✓ | ✓ | Prevent deficiencies, toxicity | |
| Electrolytes | ✓ | ✓ | ✓ | | |
| • Anthropometrics Weight, height, LBM, BCM | ✓ | ✓ | ✓ | Minimize weight loss, minimize LBM and BCM loss | Maintain weight to ≥ 95% UBW, LBM, and BCM to baseline |
| • Clinical signs and symptoms | | | | Prevent dehydration, minimize severity of side effects and treatment: diarrhea, nausea/vomiting, dysphagia, anorexia | Control of symptoms |
| • Side effects | | | | | |
| • General hydration status | ✓ | ✓ | ✓ | | |
| **Functional Outcome** Adequate nutrition | ✓ | ✓ | ✓ | Maintain po adequate to perform ADLs per Karnofsky scale Instrumental ADLs | Intake adequate to maintain self per Karnofsky scale |
| **Behavioral Outcomes** | | | | | **MNT Goals** |
| • Oral intake adequate to maintain weight | ✓ | ✓ | ✓ | • Maintains weight, LBM, BCM, and hydration | • Maintain weight, LBM, BCM, and hydration |
| • Employs food/ water safety and sanitation practices | ✓ | ✓ | ✓ | • Prevents food- and water-borne illness | • Remain free of food and water illness |
| • Consumes ↑ calorie/ protein foods/supplements and has knowledge of alternative feeding routes | ✓ | ✓ | ✓ | • Maintains weight and LBM, BCM • Minimizes symptoms | • Prevent malnutrition and/or wasting |
| • Includes/avoids foods based on side effects to medication or symptoms of infection | ✓ | ✓ | ✓ | • Minimizes side effects from meds and/or symptoms of infection | • Relieve side effects of meds and/or symptoms of infection |
| • Supplements with acceptable doses of vitamins/minerals; communicates use of questionable therapies to RD as appropriate | ✓ | ✓ | ✓ | • Avoids vitamin/mineral deficiencies, toxicity; prevents use of harmful nutritional therapies | • Maintain adequate vitamin/mineral intake |
| • Smoking/caffeine/recreational drugs | ✓ | ✓ | ✓ | • ↓or stops smoking, caffeine use or social drugs. ↑ appetite and intake of food | |
| • Alcohol | ✓ | ✓ | ✓ | • ↓ or stops alcohol intake | |
| • Exercise/activities of daily living | ✓ | ✓ | ✓ | • Participates in progressive resistance and aerobic exercise 3 x/wk, maintains LBM and BCM | |
| • Complicating factors | ✓ | ✓ | ✓ | • Reduces undesirable effects | |
| • Food access including security | ✓ | ✓ | ✓ | • Adequate food security | |

# HIV/AIDS
## Medical Nutrition Therapy Protocol

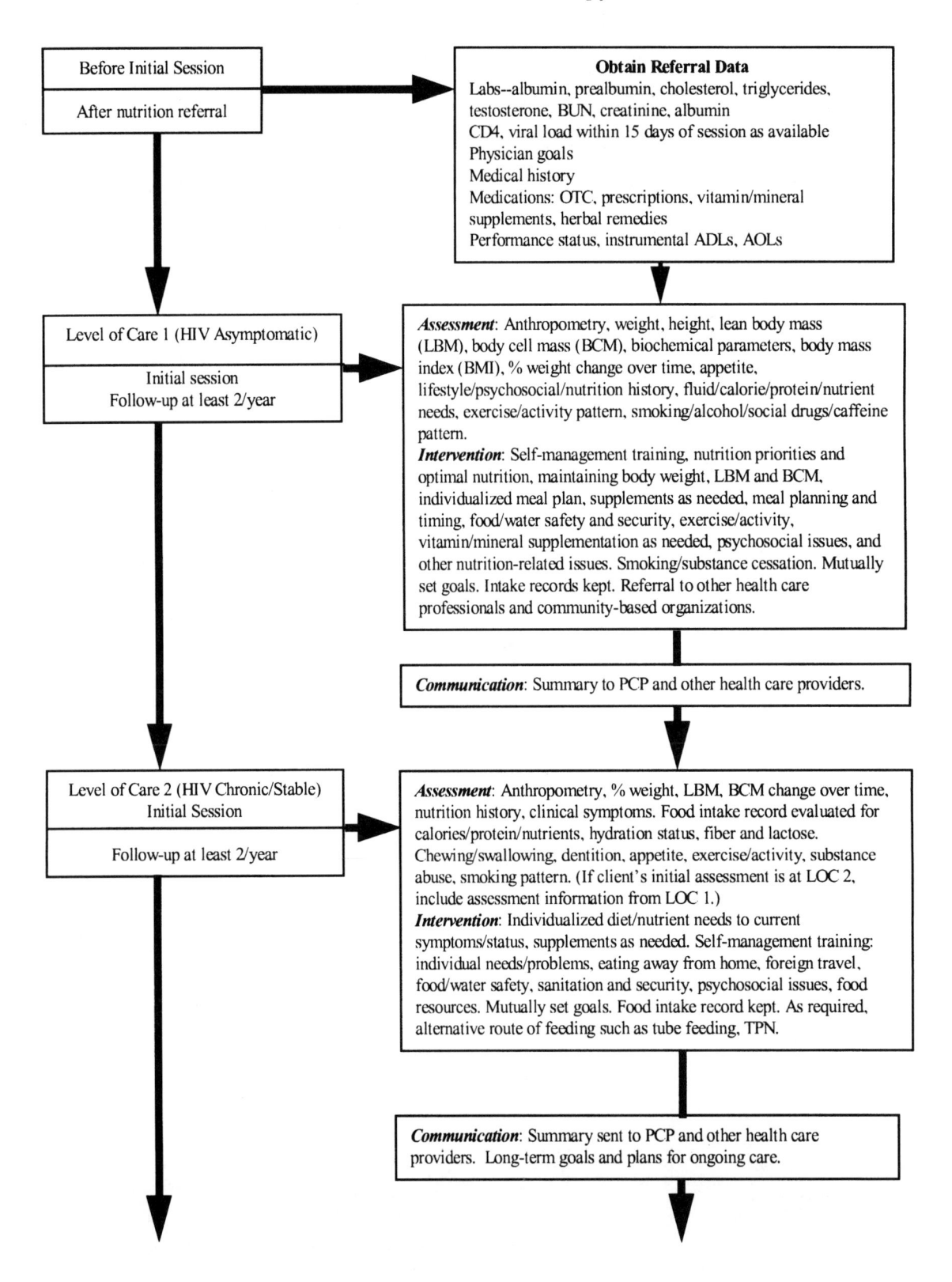

**Before Initial Session** / **After nutrition referral** →

**Obtain Referral Data**
Labs--albumin, prealbumin, cholesterol, triglycerides, testosterone, BUN, creatinine, albumin
CD4, viral load within 15 days of session as available
Physician goals
Medical history
Medications: OTC, prescriptions, vitamin/mineral supplements, herbal remedies
Performance status, instrumental ADLs, AOLs

↓

**Level of Care 1 (HIV Asymptomatic)** / Initial session / Follow-up at least 2/year →

*Assessment*: Anthropometry, weight, height, lean body mass (LBM), body cell mass (BCM), biochemical parameters, body mass index (BMI), % weight change over time, appetite, lifestyle/psychosocial/nutrition history, fluid/calorie/protein/nutrient needs, exercise/activity pattern, smoking/alcohol/social drugs/caffeine pattern.

*Intervention*: Self-management training, nutrition priorities and optimal nutrition, maintaining body weight, LBM and BCM, individualized meal plan, supplements as needed, meal planning and timing, food/water safety and security, exercise/activity, vitamin/mineral supplementation as needed, psychosocial issues, and other nutrition-related issues. Smoking/substance cessation. Mutually set goals. Intake records kept. Referral to other health care professionals and community-based organizations.

*Communication*: Summary to PCP and other health care providers.

↓

**Level of Care 2 (HIV Chronic/Stable)** Initial Session / Follow-up at least 2/year →

*Assessment*: Anthropometry, % weight, LBM, BCM change over time, nutrition history, clinical symptoms. Food intake record evaluated for calories/protein/nutrients, hydration status, fiber and lactose. Chewing/swallowing, dentition, appetite, exercise/activity, substance abuse, smoking pattern. (If client's initial assessment is at LOC 2, include assessment information from LOC 1.)

*Intervention*: Individualized diet/nutrient needs to current symptoms/status, supplements as needed. Self-management training: individual needs/problems, eating away from home, foreign travel, food/water safety, sanitation and security, psychosocial issues, food resources. Mutually set goals. Food intake record kept. As required, alternative route of feeding such as tube feeding, TPN.

*Communication*: Summary sent to PCP and other health care providers. Long-term goals and plans for ongoing care.

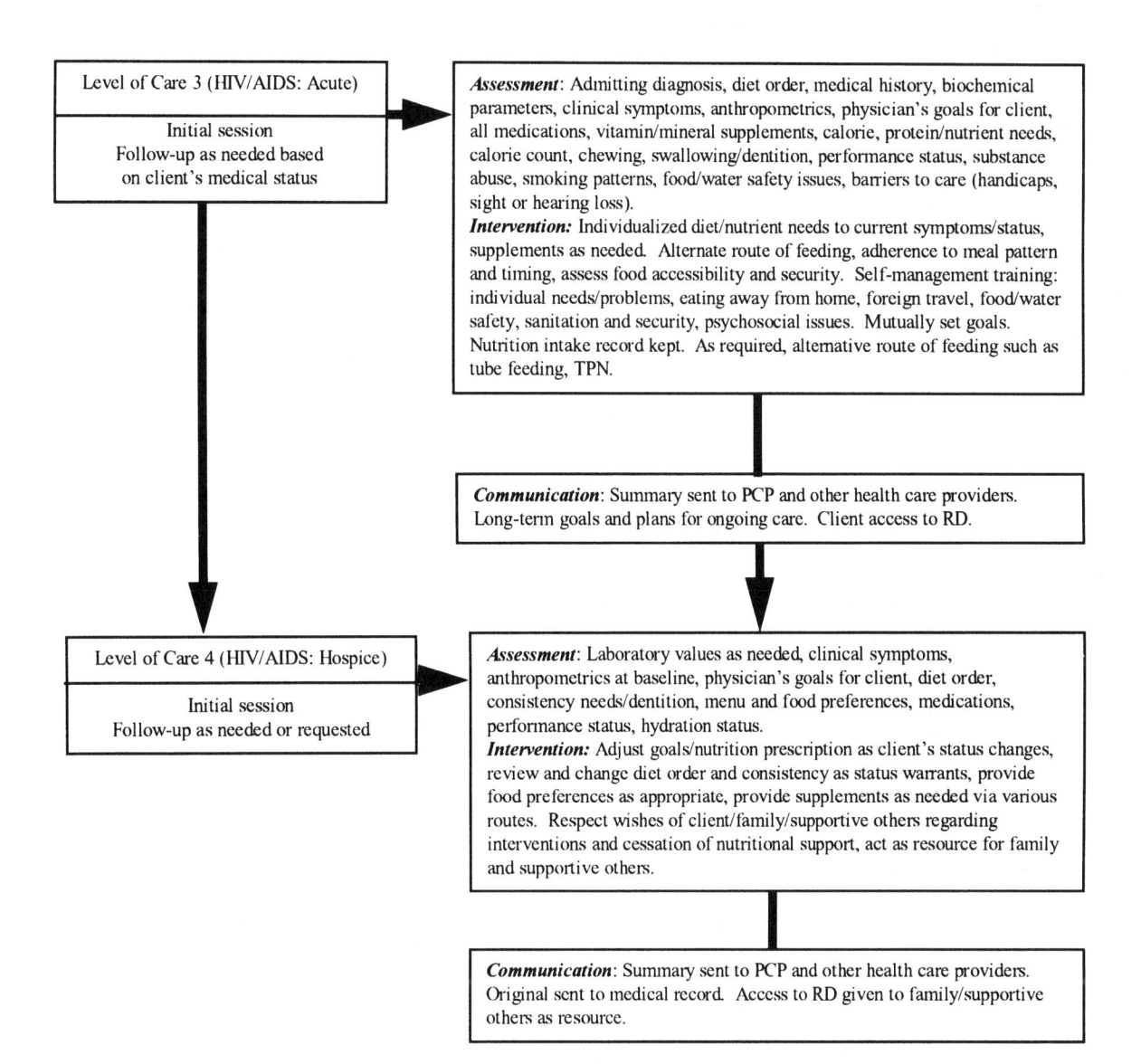

**Level of Care 3 (HIV/AIDS: Acute)**

Initial session
Follow-up as needed based on client's medical status

→ *Assessment*: Admitting diagnosis, diet order, medical history, biochemical parameters, clinical symptoms, anthropometrics, physician's goals for client, all medications, vitamin/mineral supplements, calorie, protein/nutrient needs, calorie count, chewing, swallowing/dentition, performance status, substance abuse, smoking patterns, food/water safety issues, barriers to care (handicaps, sight or hearing loss).
*Intervention:* Individualized diet/nutrient needs to current symptoms/status, supplements as needed. Alternate route of feeding, adherence to meal pattern and timing, assess food accessibility and security. Self-management training: individual needs/problems, eating away from home, foreign travel, food/water safety, sanitation and security, psychosocial issues. Mutually set goals. Nutrition intake record kept. As required, alternative route of feeding such as tube feeding, TPN.

↓

*Communication*: Summary sent to PCP and other health care providers. Long-term goals and plans for ongoing care. Client access to RD.

↓

**Level of Care 4 (HIV/AIDS: Hospice)**

Initial session
Follow-up as needed or requested

→ *Assessment*: Laboratory values as needed, clinical symptoms, anthropometrics at baseline, physician's goals for client, diet order, consistency needs/dentition, menu and food preferences, medications, performance status, hydration status.
*Intervention:* Adjust goals/nutrition prescription as client's status changes, review and change diet order and consistency as status warrants, provide food preferences as appropriate, provide supplements as needed via various routes. Respect wishes of client/family/supportive others regarding interventions and cessation of nutritional support, act as resource for family and supportive others.

↓

*Communication*: Summary sent to PCP and other health care providers. Original sent to medical record. Access to RD given to family/supportive others as resource.

PCP=primary care provider

## HIV: Level of Care 1; Asymptomatic

**Session/length: #1 for 60 minutes**

**Session Process**

*Assessment*

A. Obtain clinical data.
   1. Laboratory values with dates: albumin, prealbumin, CBC, BUN, creatinine, electrolytes, cholesterol, triglycerides, CD4, viral load, testosterone (free and total)
   2. Clinical symptoms: fever/sweats, early satiety, dysphagia, abnormal bowel habits (check for malabsorption), appetite status, dentition, lean body mass (LBM), body cell mass (BCM)
   3. Measured height and weight
   4. Physician's goals for client, health care plan and nutrition management
   5. Medical history: diabetes, cardiovascular diseases, renal disease, GI abnormalities, pancreatitis, liver disease, opportunistic infections, hepatitis
   6. All medications: over-the-counter, prescription, herbal supplements
   7. Vitamin/mineral supplements
   8. Performance status: instrumental activities of daily living (IADLs), activities of daily living (ADLs)
   9. General hydration status
   10. Questionable therapies used or being considered.

B. Interview client.
   1. Clinical data: current height/weight, body mass index (BMI), % ideal and usual weight, % weight loss over time, bioelectrical impedance assessment (BIA) and/or skinfold measurements (tricep skinfold and midarm muscle circumference), clinical symptoms (diarrhea, nausea, anorexia, and others)
   2. Nutrition history: usual food intake with attention to calories, fat, protein, lactose, and fiber content, weight history, use of vitamin/mineral/herbal supplements, over-the-counter drugs, alcohol and caffeine intake, food and water safety, and sanitation practices
   3. Exercise pattern: types of activity, frequency, and duration
   4. Psychosocial and economic issues: living situation, cooking facilities, finances, educational background, literacy level, language spoken, employment, ethnic or religious belief considerations, family support, substance abuse, food assistance (if applicable)
   5. Knowledge/readiness to learn basic nutrition principles, attitude
   6. Barriers to care: handicaps, including blindness, hearing loss, impaired language and mental functioning
   7. Smoking history: years smoked, packs presently smoked, present pattern, cessation or participation in smoking cessation program

*Intervention*

A. Adjust goals/nutrition prescription based upon assessment.
   Review records, evaluate client's adherence and understanding, and provide feedback on
   - Any HIV-related symptoms that are occurring
   - Emphasis on adequate nutrition to maintain optimal nutrition status
   - Rationale for maintaining body weight and maintaining lean body mass (LBM) and body cell mass (BCM)
   - Importance of progressive resistance training as well as aerobic exercise

- Strategies to ensure that adequate calories, protein, fat are included in diet, adherence to optimal meal plan and timing schedule to enhance drug effectiveness
- Importance of avoiding vitamin/mineral deficiencies and toxicities
- Rationale for avoiding harmful nutritional therapies
- Evaluation of need for medical nutrition supplements to provide appropriate nutrition
- Food and water safety and sanitation. Include information on water supply and other sources of cryptosporidium, giardia, and others to minimize risk of food-borne infection.
- Psychosocial issues such as support structure.
- Over-the-counter drugs, alcohol, cigarettes, and caffeine
- Potential food-drug interactions, medications, meal intake and timing.
- Setting and working on agreed-upon reasonable goals for meal planning
- Ways to record food intake and its importance in treatment
- Referral to appropriate community organizations or other health care providers

B. Provide self-management training and material on identified goals/nutrition prescription, including
  1. Goals of nutrition therapy
  2. Education materials containing information on
     - Individualized meal plans
     - Symptom management
     - Food Guide Pyramid or other healthy eating guidelines
     - Food and water safety and sanitation
     - Food intake record
     - Potential food-drug interactions
     - Community resources for food and other needs
  3. *Expected Outcome*
     - Works toward reasonable goals set with dietitian, such as improved eating habits, safe food-handling practices, supplementing diet with vitamins/minerals, meal plans, and timing as appropriate to drug regime.
     - Takes steps to alleviate related side effects, symptoms.
     - Takes measures to ensure safe water and food consumption.
     - Manages weight and preserves LBM and BCM.
     - Replenishes or preserves nutritional parameters.
     - Verbalizes understanding of potential food-drug interactions.
     - Has positive impact on quality of life, as indicated from IADL and ADL instruments.
  4. Document on Nutrition Progress Notes and other appropriate documents.

C. Follow up.
  1. Schedule appointment as determined by protocol.
  2. *Expected Outcome*
     - Works toward goal(s) set with dietitian.
     - Takes steps to alleviate HIV and other nutrition-related symptoms.
     - Maintains weight and nutritional status, and alleviates symptoms by changing dietary intake as needed.

***Communication***
1. Instruct client to call with questions, concerns.
2. Send copy of Initial Assessment, Nutrition Progress Notes, and other appropriate documents to referral source and primary care provider as soon as possible.
3. Send original to client's medical record.
4. Contact client 24-48 hours prior to next appointment.
5. Follow up on any referrals made to ensure that contact was made and that recommendations were followed. Document results of any referrals made in client's medical record.

## HIV/AIDS: Level of Care 2; Chronic/Stable

**Session/length: # 1 for 60 minutes**

**Session Process**

*Assessment*
A. Obtain clinical data.
   1. Current weight and % change over time
   2. Food intake record kept by client
   3. Laboratory values, as available
   4. Clinical symptoms: fever/sweats, early satiety, bowel habits (check for malabsorption), appetite status, difficulty chewing or swallowing, dentition, lean body mass (LBM), body cell mass (BCM)
   5. Current medications: prescription, over-the-counter, herbal, other
   6. Current exercise pattern and type
   7. Medical status
   8. Hydration status
   9. Questionable therapies used or being considered

B. Interview client.
   1. Clinical data: current height/weight, BMI, % of ideal and usual weight, % weight loss over time, bioelectrical impedance assessment (BIA) if appropriate, and/or skinfold measurements (tricep skinfold and midarm circumference), clinical symptoms (diarrhea, nausea, anorexia, and others), history of eating disorders
   2. Nutrition history: usual food intake with attention to calories, fat, protein, lactose, and fiber content, use of vitamin/mineral/herbal supplements, over-the-counter drugs, alcohol and caffeine intake, food and water safety and sanitation practices
   3. Exercise pattern: types of activity, frequency, and duration
   4. Psychosocial and economic issues: living situation, cooking facilities, finances, educational background, literacy level, language spoken, employment, ethnic or religious belief considerations, family support, substance abuse, food assistance (if applicable)
   5. Knowledge/readiness to learn nutrition principles, attitude
   6. Barriers to care: handicaps, including blindness, hearing loss, impaired language or mental functioning
   7. Smoking history: years smoked, packs presently smoked, present patterns, cessation or participant in smoking cessation program

*Outcome Measurements:* change in client's
- Weight, LBM, and BCM
- Food intake record
- Laboratory values
- Medication interactions
- Exercise/activity pattern or activities of daily living
- Drug, caffeine, alcohol, and smoking pattern
- HIV-related and other symptoms

*Intervention*

A. Adjust goals/nutrition prescription.
   *Note: For people presenting initially, incorporate goals and nutrition prescription from Level of Care 1: Asymptomatic as appropriate.*
   Review records, evaluate client's adherence and understanding, and provide feedback on
   - Food/meal plan: calories, protein, fat, carbohydrates, fluids, and other nutrients
   - Adherence to food/meal plan and timing schedule to enhance drug efficiency
   - Exercise/activities of daily living
   - Smoking (packs/day/year), drug, caffeine, and alcohol consumption patterns

B. Provide self-management training and material as appropriate.
   1. Changes in client's status: weight, laboratory values, and clinical symptoms
   2. Importance of adequate nutrition to maintain optimal nutritional status
   3. Rational for maintaining body weight, LBM, and BCM
   4. Basic nutrition: adequate calories, other nutrients for individual nutritional needs
   5. Importance of progressive resistance training, as well as aerobic exercise, as appropriate
   6. Food and water safety and sanitation: home, eating away from home, and foreign travel
   7. Supplements as needed. Select supplements according to symptoms, such as 1 kcal/cc standard formula vs MCT-based formula. Consider incorporating modular formulas.
   8. Alternative feeding routes such as tube feeding or TPN, as indicated
   9. Strategies to ensure inclusion of adequate calories/protein/fat in diet, adherence to optimal meal plan and timing schedule to enhance drug effectiveness
   10. Access to food resources and food security
   11. Rationale and benefits of appetite stimulants, inflammatory and hormonal modulators, such as testosterone as appropriate
   12. Food and water safety and sanitation. Include information on water supply and other sources of cryptosporidium, giardia, etc, to minimize risk of food/water-borne infection.
   13. Psychosocial issues and support
   14. Over-the-counter drugs, alcohol, cigarettes, and caffeine
   15. Potential food/drug interactions, medications, meal intake and timing
   16. Setting and working on reasonable goals for meal planning and other issues
   17. Ways to record food intake record and its importance in treatment
   18. Referral to appropriate community organizations or other health care providers
   19. Documentation on Nutrition Progress Notes and other appropriate documentation

*Expected Outcome*
- Works toward reasonably set goals with dietitian, such as improved eating habits, safe food-handling practices, supplementation with vitamins/minerals, and adherence to meal plans and timing as appropriate to drug regimen.
- Takes steps to alleviate related side effects/symptoms.
- Completes food intake record.
- Manages weight and preserves LBM and BCM.
- Replenishes or preserves nutritional parameters.
- Verbalizes understanding of potential food/drug interactions.
- Has positive impact on quality of life, as indicated from instrument used.

C. Follow up.
   1. At least 2-6 times per year per protocol
   2. *Expected Outcome*
      - Takes steps to alleviate HIV and other nutrition-related symptoms.
      - Completes food intake record.
      - Maintains weight and nutritional status by changing dietary intake as needed.

### *Communication*
1. Instruct client to call RD with questions/concerns.
2. Send copy of Nutrition Progress Notes and other appropriate documents to referral source and primary care provider.
3. Send original to client's medical record.
4. Contact client 24-48 hours prior to next appointment.
5. Follow up on any referrals made to ensure that contact was made and that recommendations were followed. Document results of any referrals made in client's medical record.

## HIV/AIDS: Level of Care 3; Acute

**Session/length:** As needed based on client's medical status and need

**Session Process**

*Assessment*

A. Obtain clinical data.
   1. Admitting diagnosis
   2. Medical history: diabetes, cardiovascular disease, renal disease, GI abnormalities, opportunistic infections, pancreatitis, liver disease, hepatitis
   3. Laboratory values with dates: albumin, prealbumin, CBC, BUN, creatinine, electrolytes, cholesterol, triglycerides, CD4, viral load, testosterone (free and total), as available
   4. Clinical symptoms: fever/sweats, early satiety, appetite changes, dysphagia, abnormal bowel patterns (check for malabsorption), dentition
   5. Measured height and current weight, weight changes, goal weight, BMI, LBM, BCM
   6. Physician's goals for client
   7. All medications: over-the-counter, prescription, herbal, other
   8. Vitamin/mineral supplements
   9. Performance status: instrumental activities of daily living
   10. General hydration status
   11. Calorie count, if appropriate
   12. Barriers to intake, food accessibility after visit

B. Interview client.
   1. Clinical data: current height/weight, BMI, % ideal and usual weight, % weight loss over time, bioelectrical impedance assessment (BIA) if appropriate, or skinfold measurements (tricep skinfold and midarm muscle circumference), clinical symptoms (diarrhea, nausea, anorexia, and others), history of eating disorders
   2. Nutrition history: usual food intake with attention to calories, fat, protein, lactose, and fiber content, weight history, use of vitamin/mineral/herbal supplement, over-the-counter drugs, alcohol and caffeine intake, food and water safety and sanitation practices
   3. Exercise pattern: type of activity, frequency, and duration
   4. Psychosocial and economic issues: living situation, cooking facilities, finances, educational background, literacy level, language spoken, employment, ethnic or religious belief considerations, family support, substance abuse, food assistance (if applicable)
   5. Knowledge/readiness to learn nutrition principles, attitude
   6. Barriers to care: handicaps, including blindness, hearing loss, impaired language or mental functioning
   7. Smoking history: years smoked, packs presently smoked, present patterns, cessation or participation in smoking cessation program

*Outcome Measurements:* change in client's
- Weight, LBM, BCM
- Nutrition intake
- Laboratory values
- Medications
- Exercise/activity pattern or activities of daily living

- Drug, caffeine, alcohol, and smoking patterns
- HIV and related symptoms

### *Intervention*

A. Adjust goals/nutrition prescription.

   *Note: For people presenting initially, incorporate goals and nutrition prescription from Level of Care 1: Asymptomatic and 2: Chronic/Stable as appropriate.*

   Review records, evaluate client's adherence and understanding, and provide feedback.
   - Review diet order, make recommendations to provider as appropriate.
   - Check for adherence to food/meal plan and timing schedule to enhance drug efficiency, especially if patient is hospitalized.
   - Assess exercise/activities of daily living.
   - Assess food accessibility, refer to community organizations and other health care providers as necessary and appropriate.
   - Evaluate smoking (packs/day/year), drug, caffeine, alcohol consumption patterns.
   - Provide PCP with feedback, nutrition-related recommendations for client.

B. Provide self-management training and material as appropriate on
   1. Meal planning, meal content, and timing as appropriate for diagnosis and medications
   2. Appropriate supplements as needed. Select supplements according to symptoms such as 1 kcal/cc standard formula vs MCT-based formula. Consider incorporation of modular formula.
   3. Care and management of alternate feeding routes, such as tube feeding or TPN as needed
   4. Change in weight status, laboratory values, and clinical symptoms
   5. Importance of adequate nutrition to maintain optimal nutritional status
   6. Basic nutrition: adequate calories/nutrients for individual nutritional needs
   7. Food and water safety and sanitation: home, eating away from home, and foreign travel
   8. Resources for access to food and food security information
   9. Potential food/drug interactions, medications, meal intake and timing
   10. Tip sheets on related symptom and side effect management
   11. Document on Nutrition Progress Notes and other appropriate documents.

### *Expected Outcome*

- Works toward reasonably set goals with dietitian, such as improved eating habits and food/water safety, meal planning and timing as appropriate to drug therapy.
- Takes steps to alleviate related side effects/symptoms.
- Completes nutritional intake record.
- Manages weight and preserves LBM and BCM.
- Replenishes or preserves nutritional parameters.
- Has positive impact on quality of life, as indicated from instrument used.
- Verbalizes potential food/drug interactions.

C. Follow up.
   1. Schedule follow-up with dietitian within 2 weeks after discharge.
   2. *Expected Outcomes*
      - Works toward goals mutually agreed upon with dietitian.
      - Takes steps to alleviate HIV and other nutrition-related symptoms.

- Maintains weight, nutritional status, and alleviates symptoms by changing dietary intake as needed.

### *Communication*
1. Instruct client to call with questions/concerns.
2. Send copy of Nutrition Progress Notes and other appropriate documents to referral source and primary care provider.
3. Send original to client's medical record.
4. Contact PCP or attending physician to discuss recommendations regarding nutritional status.
5. Contact other health care providers as needed to address barriers to nutritional intake.
6. Follow up on any referral made to ensure that contact was made and that recommendations were followed. Document results of any referrals made in client's medical record.

## HIV/AIDS: Level of Care 4: Hospice

**Session/length: Scheduled as needed**

**Session Process**

*Assessment*
A. Obtain clinical data.
   1. Laboratory values as needed
   2. Clinical symptoms as appropriate
   3. Measured height and weight, baseline and amount
   4. Physician's goals for client
   5. Diet order/consistancy needs/dentition
   6. Menu and food preferences/allergies
   7. All medications: over-the-counter, prescription, and herbal supplements
   8. Performance status: ADLs or IADLs
   9. General hydration status

B. Interview client/family/support givers.
   1. Menu and food preferences/allergies
   2. Food consistency needs
   3. HIV and other nutritionally related symptoms
   4. Performance status: ADLs, IADLs, and mental functioning
   5. Nutritional concerns of family members
   6. Barriers to care: handicaps, including blindness, hearing loss, impaired language and mental functioning
   7. Wishes regarding continued nutrition/hydration support

*Outcome Measurements*: change in client's
   - Comfort and quality of life
   - Hydration status
   - HIV and other nutrition-related symptoms

***Intervention***
A. Adjust goals/nutrition prescription as client's status changes.
   - Review diet order/change diet order and consistency as status warrants.
   - Provide food preferences as appropriate.
   - Provide supplements as needed via various routes.
   - Respect wishes of client/family/supportive others for level of nutrition intervention.
   - Act as resource for family and supportive others.
   - Document in Nutrition Progress Notes and other appropriate documents.

B. Provide staff, family, supportive others training and material as appropriate on
   1. Management of HIV/AIDS-related symptoms that are occurring
   2. Physician's goals for client
   3. Diet order and food consistency needs
   4. Menu and food preferences, allergies, intolerances
   5. Medications and supplement usage

6. Possible food-drug interactions
7. Keeping client hydrated as appropriate
8. Overcoming barriers to care: handicaps, including blindness, hearing loss, language problems
9. Providing PCP with feedback, nutrition-related recommendations for client as appropriate
10. Wishes regarding continued nutrition, hydration status
11. Documentation in Nutrition Progress Notes and other appropriate documents

*Expected Outcome*
- Symptoms are relieved as much as possible.
- Diet order and consistency needs are met.
- Food preferences, intolerances, and allergies are considered.
- Food-drug interactions are addressed as appropriate.
- Barriers to care are overcome as appropriate.
- Wishes are upheld regarding client's nutrition, hydration status.
- Documentation is made in Nutrition Progress Notes and other appropriate documents.

C. Follow up.
1. Schedule follow-up with dietitian as needed.
2. *Expected Outcomes*
   - Desired meal plan/diet order/food preferences and consistancy for client are met.
   - Supplements are provided as needed.
   - Takes steps to alleviate HIV and other nutrition-related symptoms.
   - Wishes of client and family regarding level of nutrition intervention met.

*Communication*
1. Instruct client/family/support givers to call with questions or concerns.
2. Send copy of Nutrition Progress Notes and other appropriate documents to referral source and primary care provider.
3. Send original to client's medical record.
4. Contact PCP or attending physician to discuss recommendations regarding nutritional status.
5. Follow up on any recommendations made.

# Appendix B: Nutrition Assessment

**NUTRITION PROGRESS NOTES**
**HIV/AIDS**
**Other Diagnosis:** _____

Level of Care   1   2   3   4

Patient's Name: _____
Medical Record #: _____
Referring Physician: _____
Primary Care Provider: _____
Language: Spoken____ Written____ Read____

## Outcomes of Medical Nutrition Therapy (MNT)

| Expected Outcome | Intervention provided to meet goal (Intervention = self-management training plus patient verbalizes/demonstrates) ||| Goal reached (Check indicates goal reached) |||
|---|---|---|---|---|---|---|
| Date / Session | 1 (60 min) | 2 (30 min) | 3 (30 min) | 1 | 2 | 3 |
| **Clinical Outcomes**<br>  Albumin<br>  Prealbumin<br>  HgB<br>  Hct<br>  Cholesterol<br>  Triglycerides<br>  BUN<br>  Creatinine<br>  CD4<br>  Viral load<br>  Height ____ Weight (goal____)<br>  Measured IBW/UBW<br>  Lean body mass (LBM)<br>  Body cell mass<br>Other_____ | | | | Value<br>____mg/dL<br>____mg/dL<br>____g/dL<br>____vol%<br>____mg/dL<br>____mg/dL<br>____mg/dL<br>____mg/dL<br><br><br>____lb<br><br><br> | Value<br>____mg/dL<br>____mg/dL<br>____g/dL<br>____vol%<br>____mg/dL<br>____mg/dL<br>____mg/dL<br>____mg/dL<br><br><br>____lb<br><br><br> | Value<br>____mg/dL<br>____mg/dL<br>____g/dL<br>____vol%<br>____mg/dL<br>____mg/dL<br>____mg/dL<br>____mg/dL<br><br><br>____lb<br><br><br> |
| **MNT Goal—Est needs**<br>• Kcal_____<br>• Protein (g)_____<br>• Fluid (oz)_____<br>• Fat (g)_____ | | | | %____kcal<br>%____g pro<br>%__oz fluid<br>%____fat<br>____meals<br>____snacks | %____kcal<br>%____g pro<br>%__oz fluid<br>%____fat<br>____meals<br>____snacks | %____kcal<br>%____g pro<br>%__oz fluid<br>%____fat<br>____meals<br>____snacks |
| **Functional Outcome:**<br>  Karnofsky or ECOG performance scale | | | | | | |
| **Behavioral Outcomes**<br>• Maintains hydration<br>• Prevents food/water-borne illnesses<br>• Consumes high-calorie/protein foods as prescribed<br>• Consumes/avoids foods that lessen side effects of infection/meds<br>• Uses acceptable nutrition therapies<br>• ↓ or stops smoking<br>• Participates in resistance/aerobic exercise 3x/wk<br>• Verbalizes potential food/drug interaction<br><br>Drug_____ | | | | <br><br><br><br><br><br><br>____ppd<br>____x/wk<br><br><br><br>____dose<br>____dose | <br><br><br><br><br><br><br>____ppd<br>____x/wk<br><br><br><br>____dose<br>____dose | <br><br><br><br><br><br><br>____ppd<br>____x/wk<br><br><br><br>____dose<br>____dose |
| **Overall Compliance Potential**<br>• Comprehension<br>• Receptivity<br>• Adherence | | | | E G P<br>E G P<br>E G P | E G P<br>E G P<br>E G P | E G P<br>E G P<br>E G P |

## B-2  Walter Reed Staging Classification for HIV Infection[a]

| Stage | HIV Status | Chronic Lymphadenopathy | CD4 Cells/mm$^3$ | Delayed Cutaneous Hypersensitivity | Thrush | OI |
|---|---|---|---|---|---|---|
| WR0 | − | Possible exposure | >400 | Normal | 0 | 0 |
| WR1 | + | 0 | >400 | Normal | 0 | 0 |
| WR2 | + | + | >400 | Normal | 0 | 0 |
| WR3 | + | ± | <400 | Normal | 0 | 0 |
| WR4 | + | ± | <400 | Partial loss | 0 | 0 |
| WR5 | + | ± | <400 | Complete loss and/or thrush | + | 0 |
| WR6 | + | ± | <400 | Partial or complete loss | ± | + |

Source: Redfield RR, Wright DC, Tramont EC. The Walter Reed staging classification for HTLV-III/LAV infection. *N Engl J Med.* 1984;314:131-132. Reproduced with permission.

[a] OI indicates opportunistic infection; minus sign, negative; plus sign, positive; zero, absent; and plus-or-minus sign, present or not present.

## B-3  Karnofsky Scale of Performance Status

| | | |
|---|---|---|
| Able to carry on normal activity; no special care is needed | 100 | Normal; no complaints; no evidence of disease |
| | 90 | Able to carry on normal activity; minor signs or symptoms of disease |
| | 80 | Normal activity with effort; some signs or symptoms of disease |
| Unable to work; able to live at home and care for most personal needs; a varying amount of assistance is needed | 70 | Cares for self; unable to carry on normal activity or to do active work |
| | 60 | Requires occasional assistance but is able to care for most needs |
| | 50 | Requires considerable assistance and frequent medical care |
| Unable to care for self; requires equivalent of institutional or hospital care; disease may be progressing rapidly | 40 | Disabled; requires special care and assistance |
| | 30 | Severely disabled; hospitalization is indicated although death is not imminent |
| | 20 | Very sick; hospitalization necessary; active supportive treatment is necessary |
| | 10 | Moribund, fatal processes progressing rapidly |
| | 0 | Dead |

Source: Sanford JP, Sande MA, Gilbert DN, Gerberding JL. *The Sanford Guide to HIV/AIDS Therapy.* Dallas, Tex: Antimicrobial Therapy, Inc; 1994. Reprinted with permission.

## B-4 Standardized Methods for Measuring Height and Weight

### HEIGHT

1. Ask the subject to stand with his or her back against the wall and with heels together.
2. Heels, scapula, and buttocks should touch the wall.
3. Chin should be tucked in and the subject encouraged to stretch to full height.
4. Using a right-angle headboard, note the height at the crown of the subject's head.

### WEIGHT

1. Calibrate the scale.
2. Ask the subject to stand without moving on the scale.
3. Record weight to 1/4 lb after scale has stabilized.
4. Weigh twice; two consecutive measurements should agree within 0.1 kg or 1/4 lb.

## B-5 Body Mass Index Values

| Height (in) | 100 | 110 | 120 | 130 | 140 | 150 | 160 | 170 | 180 | 190 | 200 |
|---|---|---|---|---|---|---|---|---|---|---|---|
| 60 | 19.6 | 21.5 | 23.5 | 25.4 | 27.4 | 29.4 | 31.3 | 33.3 | 35.2 | 37.2 | 39.1 |
| 61 | 18.9 | 20.8 | 22.7 | 24.6 | 26.5 | 28.4 | 30.3 | 32.2 | 34.1 | 36.0 | 37.9 |
| 62 | 18.3 | 20.2 | 22.0 | 23.8 | 25.7 | 27.5 | 29.3 | 31.2 | 33.0 | 34.8 | 36.7 |
| 63 | 17.8 | 19.5 | 21.3 | 23.1 | 24.9 | 26.6 | 28.4 | 30.2 | 32.0 | 33.7 | 35.5 |
| 64 | 17.2 | 18.9 | 20.6 | 22.4 | 24.1 | 25.8 | 27.5 | 29.2 | 31.0 | 32.7 | 34.4 |
| 65 | 16.7 | 18.3 | 20.0 | 21.7 | 23.3 | 25.0 | 26.7 | 28.3 | 30.0 | 31.7 | 33.4 |
| 66 | 16.2 | 17.8 | 19.4 | 21.0 | 22.6 | 24.3 | 25.9 | 27.5 | 29.1 | 30.7 | 32.3 |
| 67 | 15.7 | 17.3 | 18.8 | 20.4 | 22.0 | 23.5 | 25.1 | 26.7 | 28.3 | 29.8 | 31.4 |
| 68 | 15.2 | 16.8 | 18.3 | 19.8 | 21.3 | 22.9 | 24.4 | 25.9 | 27.4 | 28.9 | 30.5 |
| 69 | 14.8 | 16.3 | 17.8 | 19.2 | 20.7 | 22.2 | 23.7 | 25.2 | 26.6 | 28.1 | 29.6 |
| 70 | 14.4 | 15.8 | 17.3 | 18.7 | 20.1 | 21.6 | 23.0 | 24.4 | 25.9 | 27.3 | 28.8 |
| 71 | 14.0 | 15.4 | 16.8 | 18.2 | 19.6 | 21.0 | 22.4 | 23.8 | 25.2 | 26.6 | 28.0 |
| 72 | 13.6 | 14.9 | 16.3 | 17.7 | 19.0 | 20.4 | 21.7 | 23.1 | 24.5 | 25.8 | 27.2 |
| 73 | 13.2 | 14.5 | 15.9 | 17.2 | 18.5 | 19.8 | 21.2 | 22.5 | 23.8 | 25.1 | 26.4 |
| 74 | 12.9 | 14.2 | 15.4 | 16.7 | 18.0 | 19.3 | 20.6 | 21.9 | 23.2 | 24.4 | 25.7 |
| 75 | 12.5 | 13.8 | 15.0 | 16.3 | 17.5 | 18.8 | 20.0 | 21.3 | 22.5 | 23.8 | 25.1 |

Weight (lb)

# B-6 Anthropometric Values and Procedures

## VALUES

### A. Percentiles for Triceps Skinfold (TSF) for Whites and Blacks*

**Triceps Skinfold Thickness: White Adults, United States: 1971 to 1974**

| Age Group | n | 5 | 10 | 25 | 50 | 75 | 90 | 95 | n | 5 | 10 | 25 | 50 | 75 | 90 | 95 |
|---|---|---|---|---|---|---|---|---|---|---|---|---|---|---|---|---|
| | | | | Males | | | | | | | | Females | | | | |
| 1-1.9 | 226 | 6 | 7 | 8 | 10 | 12 | 14 | 16 | 204 | 6 | 7 | 8 | 10 | 12 | 14 | 16 |
| 2-2.9 | 223 | 6 | 7 | 8 | 10 | 12 | 14 | 15 | 208 | 6 | 8 | 9 | 10 | 12 | 15 | 16 |
| 3-3.9 | 220 | 6 | 7 | 8 | 10 | 11 | 14 | 15 | 208 | 7 | 8 | 9 | 11 | 12 | 14 | 15 |
| 4-4.9 | 220 | 6 | 6 | 8 | 9 | 11 | 12 | 14 | 208 | 7 | 8 | 8 | 10 | 12 | 14 | 16 |
| 5-5.9 | 214 | 6 | 6 | 8 | 9 | 11 | 14 | 15 | 219 | 6 | 7 | 8 | 10 | 12 | 15 | 18 |
| 6-6.9 | 117 | 5 | 6 | 7 | 8 | 10 | 13 | 16 | 118 | 6 | 6 | 8 | 10 | 12 | 14 | 16 |
| 7-7.9 | 122 | 5 | 6 | 7 | 9 | 12 | 15 | 17 | 126 | 6 | 7 | 9 | 11 | 13 | 16 | 18 |
| 8-8.9 | 117 | 5 | 6 | 7 | 8 | 10 | 13 | 16 | 118 | 6 | 8 | 9 | 12 | 15 | 18 | 24 |
| 9-9.9 | 121 | 6 | 6 | 7 | 10 | 13 | 17 | 18 | 125 | 8 | 8 | 10 | 13 | 16 | 20 | 22 |
| 10-10.9 | 146 | 6 | 6 | 8 | 10 | 14 | 18 | 21 | 152 | 7 | 8 | 10 | 12 | 17 | 23 | 27 |
| 11-11.9 | 122 | 6 | 6 | 8 | 11 | 16 | 20 | 24 | 117 | 7 | 8 | 10 | 13 | 18 | 24 | 28 |
| 12-12.9 | 153 | 6 | 6 | 8 | 11 | 14 | 22 | 28 | 129 | 8 | 9 | 11 | 14 | 18 | 23 | 27 |
| 13-13.9 | 134 | 5 | 5 | 7 | 10 | 14 | 22 | 26 | 151 | 8 | 8 | 12 | 15 | 21 | 26 | 30 |
| 14-14.9 | 131 | 4 | 5 | 7 | 9 | 14 | 21 | 24 | 141 | 9 | 10 | 13 | 16 | 21 | 26 | 28 |
| 15-15.9 | 128 | 4 | 5 | 6 | 8 | 11 | 18 | 24 | 117 | 8 | 10 | 12 | 17 | 21 | 25 | 32 |
| 16-16.9 | 131 | 4 | 5 | 6 | 8 | 12 | 16 | 22 | 142 | 10 | 12 | 15 | 18 | 22 | 26 | 31 |
| 17-17.9 | 133 | 5 | 5 | 6 | 8 | 12 | 16 | 19 | 114 | 10 | 12 | 13 | 19 | 24 | 30 | 37 |
| 18-18.9 | 91 | 4 | 5 | 6 | 9 | 13 | 20 | 24 | 109 | 10 | 12 | 15 | 18 | 22 | 26 | 30 |
| 19-24.9 | 531 | 4 | 5 | 7 | 10 | 15 | 20 | 22 | 1060 | 10 | 11 | 14 | 18 | 24 | 30 | 34 |
| 25-34.9 | 971 | 5 | 6 | 8 | 12 | 16 | 20 | 24 | 1987 | 10 | 12 | 16 | 21 | 27 | 34 | 37 |
| 35-44.9 | 808 | 5 | 6 | 8 | 12 | 16 | 20 | 23 | 1614 | 12 | 14 | 18 | 23 | 29 | 35 | 38 |
| 45-54.9 | 898 | 6 | 6 | 8 | 12 | 15 | 20 | 25 | 1047 | 12 | 16 | 20 | 25 | 30 | 36 | 40 |
| 55-64.9 | 734 | 5 | 6 | 8 | 11 | 14 | 19 | 22 | 809 | 12 | 16 | 20 | 25 | 31 | 36 | 38 |
| 65-74.9 | 1583 | 4 | 6 | 8 | 11 | 15 | 19 | 22 | 1670 | 12 | 14 | 18 | 24 | 29 | 34 | 36 |

From Frisancho AR. New norms of upper limb fat and muscle areas for assessment of nutritional status. *Am J Clin Nutr*. 1981;34:2540–2545. © *Am J Clin Nutr*, American Society for Clinical Nutrition. Reprinted with permission.

**Triceps Skinfold Thickness: Black Adults, United States: 1971 to 1974**

Triceps Skinfold Percentiles (mm²)

| Age Group | n | 5 | 10 | 15 | 25 | 50 | 75 | 85 | 90 | 95 | n | 5 | 10 | 15 | 25 | 50 | 75 | 85 | 90 | 95 |
|---|---|---|---|---|---|---|---|---|---|---|---|---|---|---|---|---|---|---|---|---|
| | **Males** | | | | | | | | | | **Females** | | | | | | | | | |
| 18-19 | 847 | 3 | 4 | 4 | 6 | 8 | 13 | 16 | 20 | 23 | 1,557 | 9 | 11 | 12 | 15 | 23 | 30 | 34 | 37 | 41 |
| 20-24 | 52 | 2 | 4 | 5 | 5 | 7 | 8 | 12 | 21 | 24 | 70 | 8 | 9 | 9 | 11 | 14 | 20 | 25 | 29 | 32 |
| 25-34 | 80 | 3 | 4 | 4 | 6 | 8 | 11 | 13 | 18 | 24 | 259 | 9 | 10 | 11 | 12 | 17 | 24 | 28 | 32 | 36 |
| 35-44 | 119 | 4 | 4 | 4 | 5 | 10 | 15 | 20 | 22 | 23 | 335 | 8 | 10 | 12 | 14 | 22 | 30 | 32 | 34 | 40 |
| 45-54 | 87 | 4 | 4 | 5 | 7 | 10 | 14 | 17 | 18 | 22 | 334 | 11 | 13 | 16 | 20 | 25 | 32 | 35 | 36 | 41 |
| 55-64 | 130 | 4 | 4 | 5 | 6 | 10 | 12 | 14 | 16 | 20 | 126 | 12 | 14 | 17 | 20 | 26 | 34 | 37 | 40 | 42 |
| 65-74 | 85 | 3 | 4 | 4 | 5 | 8 | 14 | 20 | 22 | 26 | 115 | 10 | 11 | 13 | 19 | 28 | 34 | 40 | 45 | 51 |
| | 294 | 4 | 4 | 5 | 6 | 9 | 12 | 14 | 15 | 19 | 318 | 7 | 11 | 15 | 17 | 24 | 30 | 32 | 35 | 40 |

*From the National Center for Health Statistics, Department of Health and Human Services, Health and Nutrition Examination Survey I, 1971-1974.

**B. Percentiles of Midarm Circumference and Estimated Midarm Muscle Circumference for Whites***

| Age Group | Arm Circumference (mm) |||||||| Arm Muscle Circumference (mm) ||||||||
|---|---|---|---|---|---|---|---|---|---|---|---|---|---|---|---|
| | 5 | 10 | 25 | 50 | 75 | 90 | 95 | | 5 | 10 | 25 | 50 | 75 | 90 | 95 |

**Males**

| Age Group | 5 | 10 | 25 | 50 | 75 | 90 | 95 | 5 | 10 | 25 | 50 | 75 | 90 | 95 |
|---|---|---|---|---|---|---|---|---|---|---|---|---|---|---|
| 1-1.9 | 142 | 146 | 150 | 159 | 170 | 176 | 183 | 110 | 113 | 119 | 127 | 135 | 144 | 147 |
| 2-2.9 | 141 | 145 | 153 | 162 | 170 | 178 | 185 | 111 | 114 | 122 | 130 | 140 | 146 | 150 |
| 3-3.9 | 150 | 153 | 160 | 167 | 175 | 184 | 190 | 117 | 123 | 131 | 137 | 143 | 148 | 153 |
| 4-4.9 | 149 | 154 | 162 | 171 | 180 | 186 | 192 | 123 | 126 | 133 | 141 | 148 | 156 | 159 |
| 5-5.9 | 153 | 160 | 167 | 175 | 185 | 195 | 204 | 128 | 133 | 140 | 147 | 154 | 162 | 169 |
| 6-6.9 | 155 | 159 | 167 | 179 | 188 | 209 | 228 | 131 | 135 | 142 | 151 | 161 | 170 | 177 |
| 7-7.9 | 162 | 167 | 177 | 187 | 201 | 223 | 230 | 137 | 139 | 151 | 160 | 168 | 177 | 190 |
| 8-8.9 | 162 | 170 | 177 | 190 | 202 | 220 | 245 | 140 | 145 | 154 | 162 | 170 | 182 | 187 |
| 9-9.9 | 175 | 178 | 187 | 200 | 217 | 249 | 257 | 151 | 154 | 161 | 170 | 183 | 196 | 202 |
| 10-10.9 | 181 | 184 | 196 | 210 | 231 | 262 | 274 | 156 | 160 | 166 | 180 | 191 | 209 | 221 |
| 11-11.9 | 185 | 190 | 202 | 223 | 244 | 261 | 280 | 159 | 165 | 173 | 183 | 195 | 205 | 230 |
| 12-12.9 | 193 | 200 | 214 | 232 | 254 | 282 | 303 | 167 | 171 | 182 | 195 | 210 | 223 | 241 |
| 13-13.9 | 194 | 211 | 228 | 247 | 263 | 286 | 301 | 172 | 179 | 196 | 211 | 226 | 238 | 245 |
| 14-14.9 | 220 | 226 | 237 | 253 | 283 | 303 | 322 | 189 | 199 | 212 | 223 | 240 | 260 | 264 |
| 15-15.9 | 222 | 229 | 244 | 264 | 284 | 311 | 320 | 199 | 204 | 218 | 237 | 254 | 266 | 272 |
| 16-16.9 | 244 | 248 | 262 | 278 | 303 | 324 | 343 | 213 | 225 | 234 | 249 | 269 | 287 | 296 |
| 17-17.9 | 246 | 253 | 267 | 285 | 308 | 336 | 347 | 224 | 231 | 245 | 258 | 273 | 294 | 312 |
| 18-18.9 | 245 | 260 | 276 | 297 | 321 | 353 | 379 | 226 | 237 | 252 | 254 | 283 | 298 | 324 |
| 19-24.9 | 262 | 272 | 288 | 308 | 331 | 355 | 372 | 238 | 245 | 257 | 273 | 289 | 309 | 321 |
| 25-34.9 | 271 | 282 | 300 | 319 | 342 | 362 | 375 | 243 | 250 | 264 | 279 | 298 | 314 | 326 |
| 35-44.9 | 278 | 287 | 305 | 326 | 345 | 363 | 374 | 247 | 255 | 269 | 286 | 302 | 318 | 327 |
| 45-54.9 | 267 | 281 | 301 | 322 | 342 | 362 | 376 | 239 | 249 | 265 | 281 | 300 | 315 | 326 |
| 55-64.9 | 258 | 273 | 296 | 317 | 336 | 355 | 369 | 236 | 245 | 260 | 278 | 295 | 310 | 320 |
| 65-74.9 | 248 | 263 | 285 | 307 | 325 | 344 | 355 | 223 | 235 | 251 | 268 | 284 | 298 | 306 |

## B. Percentiles of Midarm Circumference and Estimated Midarm Muscle Circumference for Whites* (Continued)

### Females

| Age Group | Arm Circumference (mm) 5 | 10 | 25 | 50 | 75 | 90 | 95 | Arm Muscle Circumference (mm) 5 | 10 | 25 | 50 | 75 | 90 | 95 |
|---|---|---|---|---|---|---|---|---|---|---|---|---|---|---|
| 1-1.9 | 138 | 142 | 148 | 156 | 164 | 172 | 177 | 105 | 111 | 117 | 124 | 132 | 139 | 143 |
| 2-2.9 | 142 | 145 | 152 | 160 | 167 | 176 | 184 | 111 | 114 | 119 | 126 | 133 | 142 | 147 |
| 3-3.9 | 143 | 150 | 158 | 167 | 175 | 183 | 189 | 113 | 119 | 124 | 132 | 140 | 146 | 152 |
| 4-4.9 | 149 | 154 | 160 | 169 | 177 | 184 | 191 | 115 | 121 | 128 | 136 | 144 | 152 | 157 |
| 5-5.9 | 153 | 157 | 165 | 175 | 185 | 203 | 211 | 125 | 128 | 134 | 142 | 151 | 159 | 165 |
| 6-6.9 | 156 | 162 | 170 | 176 | 187 | 204 | 211 | 130 | 133 | 138 | 145 | 154 | 166 | 171 |
| 7-7.9 | 164 | 167 | 174 | 183 | 199 | 216 | 231 | 129 | 135 | 142 | 151 | 160 | 171 | 176 |
| 8-8.9 | 168 | 172 | 183 | 195 | 214 | 247 | 261 | 138 | 140 | 151 | 160 | 171 | 183 | 194 |
| 9-9.9 | 178 | 182 | 194 | 211 | 224 | 251 | 260 | 147 | 150 | 158 | 167 | 180 | 194 | 198 |
| 10-10.9 | 174 | 182 | 193 | 210 | 228 | 251 | 265 | 148 | 150 | 159 | 170 | 180 | 190 | 197 |
| 11-11.9 | 185 | 194 | 208 | 224 | 248 | 276 | 303 | 150 | 158 | 171 | 181 | 196 | 217 | 223 |
| 12-12.9 | 194 | 203 | 216 | 237 | 256 | 282 | 294 | 162 | 166 | 180 | 191 | 201 | 214 | 220 |
| 13-13.9 | 202 | 211 | 223 | 243 | 271 | 301 | 338 | 169 | 175 | 183 | 198 | 211 | 226 | 240 |
| 14-14.9 | 214 | 223 | 237 | 252 | 272 | 304 | 322 | 174 | 179 | 190 | 201 | 216 | 232 | 247 |
| 15-15.9 | 208 | 221 | 239 | 254 | 279 | 300 | 322 | 175 | 178 | 189 | 202 | 215 | 228 | 244 |
| 16-16.9 | 218 | 224 | 241 | 253 | 283 | 318 | 334 | 170 | 180 | 190 | 202 | 216 | 234 | 249 |
| 17-17.9 | 220 | 227 | 241 | 264 | 295 | 324 | 350 | 175 | 183 | 194 | 205 | 221 | 239 | 257 |
| 18-18.9 | 222 | 227 | 241 | 258 | 281 | 312 | 325 | 174 | 179 | 191 | 202 | 215 | 237 | 245 |
| 19-24.9 | 221 | 230 | 247 | 265 | 290 | 319 | 345 | 179 | 185 | 195 | 207 | 221 | 236 | 249 |
| 25-34.9 | 233 | 240 | 256 | 277 | 304 | 342 | 368 | 183 | 188 | 199 | 212 | 228 | 246 | 264 |
| 35-44.9 | 241 | 251 | 267 | 290 | 317 | 356 | 378 | 186 | 192 | 205 | 218 | 236 | 257 | 272 |
| 45-54.9 | 242 | 256 | 274 | 299 | 328 | 362 | 384 | 187 | 193 | 206 | 220 | 238 | 260 | 274 |
| 55-64.9 | 243 | 257 | 280 | 303 | 335 | 367 | 385 | 187 | 196 | 209 | 225 | 244 | 266 | 280 |
| 65-74.9 | 240 | 252 | 274 | 299 | 326 | 356 | 373 | 185 | 195 | 208 | 225 | 244 | 264 | 279 |

*From Frisancho AR. New norms for upper limb fat and muscle areas for assessment of nutritional status. *Am J Clin Nutr.* 1981; 34:2450-2545. © *Am J Clin Nutr,* American Society for Clinical Nutrition. Reprinted with permission.

## PROCEDURES

Accuracy and reliability of anthropometric measurements depend on the equipment, skill of measurer, interaction between clinician and subject, and site and orientation of the subject and equipment. All measurements are performed on the right or dominant side. The following are step-by-step instructions for performing these measurements.

### MAC (upper arm circumference):
1. Measure and mark the halfway point of upper arm length between the tip of the acromial process of the shoulder and the olecranon.
2. Ask the subject to let his or her arm hang down with the palm facing inward.
3. Draw the tape measure around and measure at the midarm mark; hold perpendicular to length of arm.
4. Make sure that the tape measure does not compress tissues and is held flush against the skin with no gaps.
5. Record measurement at metal tip to nearest millimeter.

### TSF:
1. The subject's arm should be relaxed at his or her side with palm facing inward.
2. Grasp a double thickness of fat fold approximately 1 cm from the triceps measuring site at the midarm level.
3. Gently apply calipers to the site on the posterior aspect of the arm. The skinfold should be parallel to the length of the arm.
4. Look directly at the dial and read 3 to 4 seconds after application.
5. Measure until three measurements are repeatable; record reading.
6. Open calipers before removing.

## B-7 Bioelectrical Impedance Analysis (BIA) Protocol and Report[a]

Lean tissues have been used as a prognostic indicator in patients infected with HIV. Body composition, in terms of distribution of water and fat stores, and alterations from expected values are a reflection of health status. Adequate hydration status and lean tissue (protein stores) are essential for normal functioning of organs and all body systems.

Bioelectrical impedance analysis may reflect early and subclinical changes that may precede clinical expression of infectious or other disease processes. An effective evaluation and monitoring plan will include baseline measures of BIA, weight, weight-for-height ratio, and nutrient intake analysis. Serial measurements provide data on which to establish and monitor the achievement of clinical goals.

Periodic review of BIA history can provide important insights into trends for health status. Bioelectrical impedance analysis should be performed as a part of the usual medical examination to evaluate health status and establish clinical goals for health maintenance and improve-

---
[a]See Chapter 2 for more information on interpretation of results.

ment. BIA should be used in conjunction with other clinical measures to monitor and alter treatment plans.

## STEP 1: OBTAINING AND RECORDING BIA MEASUREMENTS

All intravenous therapies should be taken into account during this measurement because BIA is a reflection of fluid stores. Electrodes are attached to the right ankle and wrist areas according to BIA instructions that accompany the machine. The machine provides a liquid crystal display (LCD) readout of resistance and reactance measures of small single-frequency electrical impulses (less than static electricity). These measures are recorded in a BIA log or other appropriate sheet for analysis by a specially designed computer software program.

Follow these steps:

1. Ask the subject to remove his or her right sock and shoe and any metal jewelry that may interfere with the test.
2. Have the subject lie on his or her back with legs parted slightly on a nonmetal surface. Place the subject's arms away from his or her sides with palms flat alongside the body.
3. Place the red-wired electrodes on the subject's hand and the black-wired electrodes on the subject's foot.
4. While the subject relaxes, turn on the BIA machine and flip the switch to the resistance setting. After the digital reading is stabilized, record the reading (it should be between 300 and 700 ohms. Alternate switch to reactance setting. After digital reading is stabilized, record the reading (it should be between 30 and 90 ohms). If digital reading does not adequately stabilize or numbers are outside the expected range, check for the proper placement and adherence of the electrodes, the subject's body movement, or any other factors that may interfere with an accurate reading.
5. Once a reading is recorded, gently remove the electrodes from the subject's hand and foot.

## STEP 2: COMPUTERIZED CALCULATION OF BODY COMPOSITION

All data are entered into the appropriate computer software program for analysis according to prompts. Special attention should be paid to the date of the test and the accuracy of data entry to ensure usable results. These data are recorded, along with sex, age, height, and current weight. Height is the most crucial anthropometric parameter and should be based on a measured height. In addition, there is space on the form to enter body type (muscular, normal, thin, obese).

## STEP 3: EVALUATION OF REPORT

The report that is generated includes entered data, an assessment of fluid status (total body water, intracellular fluid, extracellular fluid), and a nutrition assessment (basal energy needs based on the Harris-Benedict equation).

## BIA REPORT

Your bioelectrical impedance analysis report and evaluation is below.

Name: _____ Age: _____ Sex: M F (circle one)

Height: ___ inches  Weight: ___ pounds

*Resistance:* ___ ___ ___  *Reactance:* ___ ___

Body Mass Index: _____ Goal: 20-25 (less than 18 or more than 27 is associated with health risks for some people; >27 is associated with increased risk of health problems such as heart disease, high blood pressure, and diabetes)

## BIA (BIOELECTRICAL IMPEDANCE ANALYSIS)

Your BIA will tell you how well you are hydrated, how much muscle and organ tissue you have (BCM), how much bone, collagen, and fluid outside your BCM you have (ECM), as well as an estimation on your fat tissue.

Fluids (circle one):   Dehydrated   Normally hydrated   Edema

Body cell mass: _____ pounds  Goal: ____ to ____ pounds

Extracelluar mass: _____ pounds  Goal: ____ to ____ pounds

Fat: _____ pounds  Goal: ____ to ____ pounds

BCM:ECM  _____   Goal: males: >1.0; females > 0.9

Phase angle: _____   Goal: >4.8

*To accomplish your goals you may consider discussing the following with your doctor:*

_____
_____
_____
_____

Your dietary needs to maintain your current weight and function:

_____ cups of fluid each day (coffee and alcohol don't count!)

_____ calories each day

_____ grams of protein each day

| Food Group | Serving Size | Comments |
|---|---|---|
| Grains<br>____ servings | 1 slice bread, 1/2 bagel or English muffin<br>1 small tortilla, 1/2 hamburger bun<br>1/2 cup cooked rice, pasta, cereal, or potatoes<br>4-6 crackers | Good source of carbohydrate, calories, B vitamins.<br>Whole grains are a source of iron, magnesium, selenium, zinc. |
| Fruit<br>____ servings | 1/2 cup cooked or canned fruits<br>1/2 cup fruit juice<br>1 cup raw fruits* | Good source of vitamins and minerals, especially antioxidants.<br>*Follow food safety guidelines. |
| Vegetables<br>____ servings | 1/2 cup of cooked vegetables<br>1/2 cup of vegetable juice<br>1 cup raw vegetables* | Good source of vitamins and minerals, especially antioxidants.<br>*Follow food safety guidelines. |
| Dairy<br>____ servings | 8 ounces (1 cup) milk or yogurt<br>1 1/2 ounces cheese<br>1 1/2 cup frozen yogurt/ice cream | Good source of protein, B vitamins, and minerals. Use pasteurized products. |
| Protein Foods<br>____ servings | 3 ounces cooked meat, chicken, or fish<br>2 cooked eggs<br>1/2 cup nuts or tofu<br>1 cup cooked dried beans, lentils, peas | Best sources of protein, good sources of B vitamins and minerals. 3 ounces of meat is about the size of a deck of cards. |

## B-8 Methods for Measuring Hand Dynamometry

Hand dynamometer readings are conducted to test grip strength and endurance and are affected by both hydration and training. Specific methods follow:

1. Adjust the handle of the dynamometer to the subject's comfort while allowing for a good grip.
2. Record the setting on the inside gauge to set for subsequent serial measurements.
3. Set the clear plastic at the zero position before each trial.
4. Place the subject's arm at the side slightly away from the body with elbow bent (approximately 20 degrees). Ask the subject to squeeze the handle as hard as possible.
5. Administer the test to the subject's dominant and then nondominant hand.
6. Allow three trials, alternating dominant and nondominant hands, with a brief pause between trials (10 to 20 seconds). Encourage the subject to squeeze the handle as hard as possible for maximum effect.
7. Record the amount registered at each trial to the nearest whole kilogram. Note the average for each hand if scores are within 3 kg. If scores differ by more than 3 kg, repeat the test after a sufficient rest period.

# Appendix C
# Selected In-service Outlines

## In-service 1: Nutrition and Immunology

Topic: Nutrition and immune function
Length: 30 to 45 minutes
Target Audience: Clinical dietetics staff
Presenter: Clinical dietitian
Goal: To educate participants on the effect of malnutrition on immune function
Objectives: At the completion of this presentation, participants will be able to:

1. Describe the effects of malnutrition (including protein, energy, vitamin, and mineral deficits, as well as excessive nutrient intake) on the immune system
2. Critically review current research in the area of nutrition and immunology
3. Make appropriate recommendations for nutrition intervention for patients demonstrating altered immune response related to nutrition

Procedures: The dietitian will discuss:

I. Overview of the healthy immune system
   The immune system is a surveillance mechanism which provides protection from foreign substances. There are two basic types of immunity: *specific* and *nonspecific*. Both can be affected by malnutrition.

II. The immune response
    The body defends itself from antigens (foreign substances) by producing an immune response. There are two types of

immune response: *cell mediated* and *humoral*.

III. Nutrition in immunology
    A. Effects of malnutrition on the immune system
        1. Malnutrition is a primary cause of immune deficiency
        2. Mucocutaneous integrity
            a. The first barrier to a foreign substance
            b. Immunoglobulin secreted in saliva and other external body fluids is lower in malnourished children
            c. Malnutrition can lead to tissue breakdown and loss of defense
        3. Cell-mediated immunity
            a. Reduced size of thymus gland
            b. Reduced number of peripheral lymphocytes
            c. Reduced T-cell counts
            d. Anergy: delayed-type hypersensitivity
        4. Humoral immunity
            a. Less affected than cell-mediated immunity
            b. Reduced B-cell counts
    B. Immunocompetence in protein-energy malnutrition
        1. General alterations: decreased numbers and function
        2. CD4 and CD8 cell counts
        3. Delayed hypersensitivity

IV. Nutrition, immunity, and hospitalized patients
    A. Incidence of malnutrition in the hospital
        1. Occurs in 50% of severely ill patients and 24% of moderately ill patients
        2. Related to disease state and absence of nutrition support
    B. Malnutrition is associated with increased incidence of sepsis, increased morbidity, and increased mortality

V. Effects of nutritional replenishment on the immune system
    A. Many alterations in immune function can be treated with nutritional replenishment
    B. Immunoglobulin, antibody response, complement protein levels, and delayed hypersensitivity reactions will return to normal with nutrition support
    C. Summary of specific nutrients and their effect on immune function (see Table C1-1)
    D. Excess intake of nutrients and immune responses
        1. An increase in intake of either saturated or polyunsaturated fatty acids to more than 16% of kilocalories results in decreased cell-mediated immunity
        2. Slight excess of certain nutrients may be associated with enhanced immune response: beta carotene, vitamin A, vitamin E, zinc, and selenium
        3. Zinc, selenium, vitamin E, and vitamin A given at levels beyond a certain threshold will reduce immune response
        4. Excess iron may promote bacterial septicemia

VI. Immunonutrition

"Clinical nutrition therapy stands poised upon the threshold of a new era—an era in which we shall approach the goal of providing our patients with diets which maintain normal immune defenses." Charles T. Van Buren, MD

- A. Enteral nutritional products
    1. Impact (Novartis, Fremont, MI 47413)
    2. Immun-Aid (McGaw Inc, Irvine, CA 92714)
    3. Advera (Ross Laboratories, Columbus, OH 43215)
- B. Parenteral nutrition
    1. Supplemental amino acids
    2. Structured lipids

VII. Malnutrition, immunity, and the life cycle
- A. Role of breast-feeding in enhancing immune function
    1. Transfer of immune components, especially immunoglobulin A (IgA), in breast milk
    2. Reduced incidence of ear and upper airway infections as well as allergic reactions in breast-fed infants
- B. Effect of aging on immune competence
    1. Average immune function of elderly people is significantly lower than young people
    2. Correction can occur after nutritional advice and supplementation

VIII. Effect of obesity and infection with the human immunodeficiency virus (HIV) on immune function
- A. Obesity
    1. Obese adolescents and adults have higher risk of infection
    2. Impaired delayed cutaneous hypersensitivity response, decreased lymphocyte response to mitogen, and reduced bactericidal capacity of neutrophils
- B. HIV disease and the acquired immunodeficiency syndrome (AIDS) (see Table C1-2)

**Table C1-1  Summary of Nutrients and Effects on Immune Function**

| Nutrient | Proposed Effect on Immune Function |
|---|---|
| Arginine | Improved, more rapid positive nitrogen balance<br>Enhanced collagen synthesis<br>Elevated immunoglobulin, weight gain<br>Improved peripheral monocyte response to antigens and mitogen<br>Improved survival |
| Glutamine | Improved growth and repair of gut<br>Improved survival of abdominal abscess<br>Increased gut villus height and mucosal thickness<br>Lymphocyte proliferation<br>Protection of small bowel during irradiation<br>Attenuated loss of gut immune function associated with standard formulas |
| Branch chain amino acids (BCAA) | Deficiency associated with:<br>• Reduced thymic and blood lymphocytes<br>• Increased infection in animals<br>Supplementation may:<br>• Increase lymphocyte count<br>• Improve skin test reactivity |
| Tryptophan | Reduced immune response to synthetic antigen<br>Impaired phagocytosis<br>Reduced antibody production in animals |
| Essential fatty acids | Deficiency associated with:<br>• Impaired skin test reactivity<br>• Decreased humoral response to immunization<br>• Reduced cell-mediated immune response<br>N-3 polyunsaturated fatty acid supplementation may cause:<br>• Anti-inflammatory effect (reduced pro-inflammatory)<br>• Enhanced mitogenic proliferation of T and B cells |
| Vitamin A | Enhance antibody production<br>Maintain skin integrity<br>May reduce immunosuppression associated with radiation therapy<br>Enhance lymphocyte proliferation |
| Vitamin B6 | Promote cell-mediated immunity<br>Enhance lymphocyte response to mitogen and antigens<br>Enhance antibody formation past immunization |
| Vitamin C | Protect from oxidative damage<br>Enhance phagocytosis<br>Support synthesis of collagen<br>Enhance mitogen-dependent blastogenesis |
| Vitamin E | Stimulate increase in immunologic response<br>Prolong survival in irradiated animal model<br>Proliferate lymphocytes<br>Support synthesis of antibodies |
| Zinc | Deficiency associated with:<br>• Low T-cell counts and response<br>• Decreased thymic hormone activity<br>• Decreased T-cell-dependent antibody production |

**Table C1-1 Summary of Nutrients and Effects on Immune Function (Continued)**

| Nutrient | Proposed Effect on Immune Function |
|---|---|
|  | Supplementation:<br>• May reverse above immunologic deficiencies<br>• Oversupplementation associated with decreased immune function |
| Iron | Deficiency causes impaired differentiation and proliferation of precursor T cells<br>Needed by natural-killer cells, neutrophils, and lymphocytes for optimal function<br>Excess free iron may enhance bacterial growth |
| Copper | Deficiency suppresses lymphocyte function in animal model |
| Selenium | Enhance lymphocyte response in animal model<br>Act as an antioxidant |
| Nucleotides | Deficiency has been associated with:<br>• Decreased resistance to infections<br>• Delayed cutaneous hypersensitivity<br>• Delayed onset of autoimmune allergic response |

**Table C1-2 Immunologic Changes With AIDS and Protein-Energy Malnutrition**

| Roles of Immune System | AIDS | Protein-Energy Malnutrition |
|---|---|---|
| **Scavengers** |  |  |
| Neutrophils | Normal or decreased | Decreased |
| Macrophages (normal range, 56%-60% of white blood cell count) | Normal or decreased | Decreased |
| **Antibody Producers** |  |  |
| B cells | Increased | Increased |
| Capacity to recognize microbes | Decreased | Decreased |
| **Killers** |  |  |
| T8 cells | Decreased | Decreased |
| **Foremen (Coordinators)** |  |  |
| T4 cells (normal range, 800-1200/mm$^3$) | Decreased | Decreased |

Source: Cossette M. *Nutrition and HIV: Counter Attack AIDS*, Quebec, Canada: Ministère de la Santé et des Services Sociaux du Québec; 1988.

# In-service 2: Nutrition Assessment of the HIV-Positive Hospitalized Patient

Topic: Nutrition assessment of hospitalized HIV-positive patients

Length: 45 minutes

Target Audience: Clinical dietitians, dietetic technicians, nurses, physicians

Presenter: Clinical dietitian with experience in HIV-related care

Goal: To educate health care professionals on the importance and components of nutritional status assessment in HIV-positive patients

Objectives: At the completion of this in-service, participants will be able to:

1. Name the four components of nutritional status assessment
2. Identify HIV-positive patients with malnutrition or at significant risk for malnutrition
3. Describe limitations in standard nutrition assessment data associated with HIV disease
4. Describe the causes of malnutrition in HIV disease

Procedure:

The following items will be presented orally with support slides and/or written materials:

1. Nutritional status assessment form
2. Criteria for nutrition intervention
3. Nutrition screening form for hospitalized patients
4. Table C2-1: Limitations in Standard Nutrition Assessment Measures in HIV Disease

I. Screening for nutritional risk (see Chapter 2)
   A. HIV = Nutritional Risk
   B. AIDS, as defined by the Centers for Disease Control and Prevention (CDC), includes the wasting syndrome
   C. Nutrition problems commonly identified in HIV:
      1. More than 60% of patients will experience malabsorption
      2. More than 92% will experience significant weight loss
      3. More than 30% have documented vitamin or mineral deficiencies in asymptomatic stages depending on geographical location (especially for soil-based nutrients)
   D. Routine screening of hospitalized patients mandated by the Joint Commission on Accreditation of Healthcare Organizations

II. Nutritional status assessment
   A. Components
      1. Diet history
      2. Anthropometric measurements
      3. Biochemical evaluation
      4. Nutrition-oriented physical examination

B. Use
1. Routinely before initiation of specialized support
2. Regular follow-up evaluation to assess adequacy of support and adjust therapy as indicated
C. Selected limitations to standard nutritional status assessment measures in HIV disease (see Table C2-1)

III. Etiology of malnutrition in HIV disease
A. Decreased oral intake
B. Malabsorption
C. Hypermetabolism
D. Altered metabolism

IV. Criteria for nutrition intervention
A. Inpatient
1. Significant weight loss
2. Depleted visceral or somatic protein stores
3. Problems or symptoms interfering with oral intake: nausea, emesis, anorexia, early satiety, mucositis, fatigue, and so on
4. Drug-nutrient interactions
5. Indications present for specialized nutrition support
6. Newly diagnosed HIV-positive status
7. Documented malabsorption
8. Delayed wound healing
9. Chemotherapy or radiation therapy
10. Anemia or other documented nutrient deficiencies
11. Documented inadequate or limited oral intake
B. Specialized nutrition support
1. Failed oral, volitional intake
2. Significantly depleted weight
3. Significantly depleted visceral protein stores
4. Malabsorption
5. Secretory diarrhea
6. Ventilation
7. Presence of bowel parasite or AIDS-related bowel disease leading to malnutrition
8. Patient request for supplemental support

**Table C2-1 Limitations in Standard Nutrition Assessment Measures in HIV Disease**

| Nutrition Assessment Measure | Possible Limitation to Use |
|---|---|
| **Visceral Proteins** | |
| Albumin | Altered by fluid status, infection |
| Transferrin | Falsely increased with iron deficiency |
| Prealbumin | Falsely elevated with renal disease |
| **Somatic Proteins** | |
| Creatinine height index | Creatinine clearance altered in HIV |
| **Anthropometric** | |
| Weight | Altered by fluid status, does not reflect body composition |
| Triceps skinfold | Altered by fluid status |
| **Biochemical** | |
| Hemoglobin, hematocrit | Depressed in chronic disease |
| Urine urea nitrogen | Inaccurate measures with hyperproteinuria |
| Mean corpuscular volume (MCV), mean corpuscular hemoglobin concentration (MCHC) | Falsely indicate folate deficiency with zidovudine (AZT) therapy |
| **Immunologic** | |
| Skin test antigens | Anergy present with HIV disease |

## In-service 3: Medical Nutritional Products

Topic: Selecting oral medical nutritional products for the HIV-infected client
Length: 45 minutes
Audience: Registered nurses, licensed vocational nurses, pharmacists, pharmacy technicians, purchasing agents, reimbursement staff, physical therapists, occupational therapists, speech therapists
Responsibility: Dietitian
Goal: To familiarize health care providers and purchasing department and reimbursement staff to the benefits of selected medical nutritional products used in HIV disease
Objectives: At completion of this in-service, participants will be able to:

1. Recognize one product in each formula category
2. Identify three products recommended for the HIV-positive client

Procedures: The dietitian will discuss:

1. Formula categories
   a. Polymeric—milk base, lactose free
   b. Predigested—peptide based, elemental
   c. Disease specific—renal, hepatic, pulmonary, endocrine
   d. Modular—carbohydrate, protein, fat

2. Criteria for product selection for the HIV-positive client
   a. Patient preference
   b. Tolerance to lactose
   c. Volume tolerance
   d. Types of gastrointestinal (GI) symptoms
   e. Level of GI function

3. Characteristics of commonly used products in HIV
   a. Lactose containing, low cost
   b. Low fat, high protein, moderate cost
   c. Moderate fat, high MCT, high cost
   d. Peptide based, high MCT, moderate to high cost

# In-service 4: Specialized Nutrition Support in HIV Disease: Enteral Support

Topic: Enteral support in HIV disease: formula selection and monitoring
Length: 45 minutes
Audience: Nurses, pharmacists, clinical dietetics staff, physicians
Goal: To educate health care providers on the effective and appropriate use of enteral nutrition for HIV-positive patients
Objectives: At the end of this in-service, participants will be able to:

1. List two indications for use of tube feeding
2. List three aspects of monitoring tube feeding for safety and efficacy
3. Discuss characteristics of two categories of enteral formulations

Procedures:
The dietitian will discuss indications, methods, and monitoring for enteral feedings in HIV disease.

I. Purpose and characteristics of enteral feeding
   A. A tube feeding provides adequate nutrition for those who are unable to ingest enough energy orally to meet their needs.
   B. Commercial or special prepared formulas should be used.
   C. Feedings vary in adequacy depending on product and volume ordered.

II. Indications for use
   A. Physical impairments, especially oropharyngeal and esophageal
   B. Neurologic disorders
   C. Anorexia (drug, medical, or self-induced)
   D. Increased nutrient needs secondary to stress or infection
   E. Functional gastrointestinal tract even with impairment (pancreas, inflammatory bowel disease, malabsorption, low output fistula)

III. Guidelines for ordering
   A. Orders for tube feeding should include:
      1. Formula name
      2. Strength
      3. Rate
      4. Volume
      5. Time—every hour, every 4 hours (bolus), intermittent or continuous

IV. Nutrient requirements
   A. Energy: Energy requirements will vary greatly depending on the patient's age, sex, physical activity, illness, and

nutritional status.
- B. Protein: Protein requirements depend on age, sex, nutritional status, diagnosis, history of renal or hepatic disease, and nutrition history. Stress factors will increase protein requirements due to excess nitrogen losses and increased needs for tissue synthesis.
- C. Vitamins/minerals: The USDA Recommended Daily Allowances (RDA) for vitamins and minerals can be met at various kilocalorie levels depending on the commercial formula being used. Vitamin or mineral supplementation may be indicated if needs are not met by formula. Generally 1,800 mL of formula is adequate to meet the RDA.
- D. Water: Unless medically contraindicated, total fluid volume should be 30 to 35 mL/kg for adults. Newborns' fluid needs are 85 mL/kg. For infants under 3 months of age, fluid needs are 140 to 160 mL/kg; for those aged 3 months to 2 years, fluid needs are 120 mL/kg. Most enteral formulas are 75% to 85% of total fluid as free water.
- E. Osmolarity: Tube feeding should be as near to isotonic (300 mOsm/kg $H_2O$) as possible when initiated; then strength is increased as patient tolerates. Commercial feedings are generally 300 to 900 mOsm/kg $H_2O$. Diluting the strength of the formula with water reduces the osmolality.

V. Administration of enteral feeding
- A. Isotonic formulas should be started at full strength: hypertonic formulas (>400 mOsm) should be started at half strength.
- B. Although the *initial rate* of administration of feeding should be determined individually, generally a rate of 50 mL/hr will be well tolerated.
- C. After 8 hours, if tolerance is demonstrated (i.e., no nausea or vomiting, abdominal distention, or higher gastric residual), the formula may be increased in strength. Increase strength every 8 hours until full strength is obtained.
- D. After adaptation/tolerance to full strength feeding has been established, the rate of the feeding may be increased in 25- to 30-mL increments until the goal rate is obtained. *Never* increase concentration and rate simultaneously.
- E. Additional water may be administered to flush medications through the tube and/or to meet fluid requirements. Basic fluid requirements are approximately 30 to 35 mL/kg per day. Consider intravenous (IV) and oral intake as well as output to maintain balance.

VI. Principles of administration for enteral alimentation
- A. Aspirate: With nasogastric feeding, check residuals every 4 hours. With nasoduodenal feeding tubes, residuals cannot be effectively aspirated.
- B. Flush: Bolus feeding after all medications and after each feeding; continuous drip after all medications.
- C. Elevate: Raise the head of the bed at least 30 degrees dur-

ing the feeding and for 30 minutes thereafter. Stop feeding temporarily if the patient must be lowered.
- D. Slow/hold: Slow or hold the tube feeding for 2 hours when residuals are greater than 100 mL; then restart. If the residual remains significant, reduce the rate. If there is abdominal cramping or nausea, the rate of infusion should be reduced to the last tolerated rate.
- E. General considerations: If diarrhea occurs, the rate may need to be decreased. The osmolality of solutions can be reduced by diluting it with sterile water, or antidiarrheal agents may be added. Check with the pharmacist before adding medications to tube feeding formulas. Patients should be monitored daily for bowel movements, bowel sounds, or evidence of fecal impaction. Check the tube position once each shift. With a gravity drip or infusion pump, check the rate every hour. Hang no more than a 4-hour supply of formula at a time unless manufacturer's recommendations state otherwise.
- F. Monitoring enteral alimentation (see Table C4-1)

VII. Types of formulas
- A. Pediatric: Pediatric patients should be given pediatric formulas as there is not enough calcium or phosphorus in adult formulas to meet pediatric needs
- B. Isotonic: Used to minimize diarrhea, usually 1 kcal/mL (300 mOsm/kg $H_2O$). Begin isotonic formula 1 to 2 mL/kg per hour. If patient has had nothing by mouth (NPO) for more than 3 days, begin at no greater than 0.5 kcal/mL. Work up to one third to one half of the desired rate; then concentration may gradually be increased. Do not increase rate and concentration simultaneously.
- C. Elemental: Carbohydrate and protein are in simple, easier to absorb units with minimal residue. Used when patient has minimal GI function.
- D. High caloric density: Provides more than 1 kcal/mL. Used when fluid intake is limited or energy needs are exceptionally high.
- E. Disease specific: Designed to meet special needs of patients with hepatic, renal, pulmonary, diabetes, HIV, and/or other disease states according to specific types or amounts of carbohydrate, protein, fat, and/or micronutrients
- F. Fiber-containing/mixed in blender: Used to increase tolerance when intolerance to nonfiber polymeric formulas has been demonstrated
- G. Modular components: Used to increase the amount of carbohydrate, protein, or fat in a feeding

VIII. Nutritional adequacy
- A. Enteral feeding formulas are designed to provide 100% of the RDA based on a specific volume of feeding infused. Patients who have low energy requirements (elderly, immobile) may not receive 100% of their vitamin, mineral,

and trace element needs; mineral and perhaps even trace element therapy may be necessary. Also, patients on disease-specific formulas may not receive 100% of the RDA, since some of these formulas may be designed to limit specific nutrients in light of the patient's clinical condition.
B. Adult formulas may not be appropriate for children, especially infants under age 2 years, unless close attention is paid to the vitamin, mineral, and trace element adequacy. Adult formulas may also have a higher protein load than is advised in young children.
C. Practitioners are also advised to monitor the fluid status of their patients closely, especially if the patient is prescribed a fiber-containing formula.

Table C4-1  Monitoring Enteral Alimentation

| Initial or Acute Care | Long-term Care |
|---|---|
| Daily weight; intake and output | Daily weight; intake and output |
| Renal battery every day for 3 days, then every Monday and Thursday | SMAC 12 every month |
| | SMAC 20 every 3 months |
| Ca++, Mg++, phosphate every day for 2 days (or until stable), then every Monday and Thursday | White blood cell (WBC) and differential cell counts every 3 months |
| Initial albumin, transferrin, then every 2-3 weeks | Additional laboratory tests as indicated by changes in clinical condition |
| Additional laboratory tests as indicated by clinical condition | |

# In-service 5: Specialized Nutrition Support: Enteral and Parenteral Support

Topic: Specialized nutrition support (alternate in-service to enteral support)
Length: 30 to 45 minutes
Target Audience: Nursing, clinical pharmacy, physicians, clinical dietitians, and dietetic technicians
Presenter: Clinical dietitian with nutrition support expertise
Goal: To educate health care professionals on the effective and appropriate use of enteral or parenteral support in patients with HIV disease
Objectives: At the completion of this in-service, participants will be able to:

1. Identify HIV-positive clients who are potential candidates for specialized nutrition support
2. Identify and delineate the roles of specific health care professionals involved in the provision of specialized nutrition support and identify the benefits of a team approach to patient care
3. Name four goals of specialized nutrition support in patients who are HIV positive
4. Name the three general categories of enteral formulas and one indication for each; name two general bases for total parenteral formulas and one indication for each
5. Describe three common complications associated with enteral support and two common complications of parenteral support; give potential solutions for each

Procedures:
The following items will be presented orally with support slides and/or written materials:

1. Definition of enteral and parenteral support
2. Table 4-4: HIV-Related Medical Conditions That Justify Nutrition Support
3. Table 4-6: Enteral Feeding Routes and Indications
4. Review of the role and function of health professionals in the provision of nutrition support to HIV-positive persons
5. Nutrition assessment and monitoring forms

   I. Definition of terms
      A. **Enteral nutrition:** Nutrition via the gastrointestinal tract, generally referring to tube feeding
      B. **Parenteral nutrition:** Provision of nutrition support intravenously

   II. Indications for use
      A. Enteral
         1. Functional gastrointestinal tract
         2. Significant malnutrition with failure of volitional oral intake

3. Severe anorexia
4. Coma
5. Idiopathic weight loss
6. Severe dysphagia
7. Ventilation
8. Altered mental status resulting in inadequate oral intake
9. Significantly increased nutrient requirements related to illness
  B. Parenteral
1. Nonfunctional or compromised GI tract
2. AIDS enteropathy
3. Obstruction of gastrointestinal tract
4. Severe secretory diarrhea

III. Indications for use of enteral and parenteral formulas
  A. Enteral
1. Intact, polymeric: No evidence of malabsorption, normal stools, supplemental to oral nutrition
2. Elemental: Fat malabsorption, generalized malabsorption, gut which has not been used for a prolonged time (>7 days)
3. Defined formula: Mild malabsorption, presence of diarrhea, possible atrophied gut, on several medications that are known to irritate the bowel wall
4. Modular: Supplement specific components of the diet including protein, energy, fat, vitamins and minerals; used in patients with fluid restrictions and with increased energy or protein needs
  B. Parenteral
1. Dextrose-base: Normal blood glucose levels, elevated triglyceride levels, medications associated with increased lipid levels, fluid restriction
2. Fat or lipid-base: Elevated glucose levels, medications associated with glucose intolerance, patients with increased carbon dioxide production that is not attributable to overfeeding

IV. Nutritional status assessment
  A. Components
1. Diet history
2. Biochemical evaluation
3. Anthropometric measurements
4. Nutrition-oriented physical examination
  B. Use
1. Routinely before initiation of specialized support
2. Regular follow-up evaluation to assess adequacy of support and adjust therapy as indicated

V. Goals for specialized nutrition support
  A. Minimize catabolism
  B. Minimize nutrient losses

C. Replenish body cell mass
D. Improve host resistance
E. Improve pharmacologic response
F. Preserve gut function
G. Improve quality of life

VI. Health care team
   A. Why? Team approach to patient care, especially for patients receiving nutrition support, has been associated with decreased complications and improved outcome
   B. Who and what (see Table C5-1)

### Table C5-1  Role of Nutrition Support Team Members

| Team Member | Role |
| --- | --- |
| Clinical dietitian | Perform nutrition assessments; prescribe appropriate support route and therapy; monitor tolerance to therapy; communicate goals to other health care team members |
| Clinical pharmacist | Prescribe appropriate nutrition therapy; monitor impact of medications on clinical course; monitor tolerance to therapy; communicate concerns to other health care team members |
| Nurse | Administer nutrition support; monitor tolerance; monitor for nutrient-medication interactions; monitor for infection control issues; document support provided; communicate concerns to other health care team members |
| Occupational or physical therapist | Provide occupational or physical therapy as indicated; communicate care plan and concerns to other health care team members |
| Physician | Prescribe nutrition care; monitor tolerance; coordinate other professional services; communicate with other health care team members |

## In-service 6: Inpatient Nutrition and HIV Disease

Topic: Contribution of nurses to the nutrition support of HIV-infected patients
Length: 30 minutes
Audience: Registered nurses, licensed vocational nurses, and nurse's aides
Responsibility: Nurse, clinical dietitian
Goal: To establish the contributions of the nursing staff for the provision of optimal nutrition care for the HIV-infected patient
Objectives: Upon completion of this in-service, participants will be able to:

1. List at least six reasons for the development of malnutrition
2. List four actions that can be taken by the nursing staff to augment patient nutrition care

Procedure: The dietitian will discuss:

1. Causes of malnutrition
   a. Primary malnutrition: Anorexia, dysgeusia, nausea and vomiting, altered mental status, depression, food faddism, economics, dysphagia, fear of diarrhea, breathing vs eating dilemma, self-medication, pain, drug-nutrient interaction
   b. Secondary malnutrition: Increased losses from diarrhea (bowel pathogens, bacterial overgrowth, lactose intolerance), malabsorption, altered utilization or excretion (drug-nutrient interaction, stress or infectious processes, organ involvement), hormonal imbalance

2. Contribution of nursing staff to nutrition care
   a. Data collection: Intake assessment, anthropometric measurements
   b. Monitor: Change in anthropometric data, input and output, general indicators, usual parameters for enteral and parenteral nutrition, food safety
   c. Action: Obtain dietary consult, provide patient advocacy, encourage adequate intake, follow facility protocol for safety of tube feeding and total parenteral nutrition, adjust timing of medication with meals

# In-service 7: Nutrition and HIV Disease in Home Care and Hospice: Nutrition Screening

Topic: Nutrition screening in HIV disease
Length: 45 minutes
Audience: Registered nurses, licensed vocational nurses, physical therapists, occupational therapists, speech therapists
Responsibility: Dietitian
Goal: To familiarize health care providers to the role of nutritional status in HIV disease
Objectives: Upon completion of this in-service, participants will be able to:

1. Identify three factors that predispose HIV-infected clients to malnutrition
2. Identify screening tools to determine patients who would benefit from nutrition interventions
3. Identify services offered by the home health care dietitian

Procedures: The dietitian will discuss:

1. Risk factors for malnutrition
    a. Decreased intake
    b. Decreased absorption
    c. Alterations in metabolism
    d. Increased excretion

2. Physical signs of malnutrition
    a. Skin, oral cavity, hair, fingernails
    b. Reactions, cognition

3. List monitoring parameters
    a. Biochemical parameters
    b. Anthropometry
    c. Intake data
    d. Medical history
    e. Medication history

4. Referral criteria
    a. Decreased intake of food and nutrients
    b. Nausea, vomiting, constipation, diarrhea
    c. Drug-nutrient or nutrient-nutrient interactions
    d. Altered biochemical and anthropometric indexes
    e. Food faddism
    f. Inadequate food access

5. Services offered
    a. Assessment, counseling, monitoring
    b. Recommendations to physicians and staff regarding nutrition support, interactions with therapies, requested action

## In-service 8: Nutrition and HIV Disease in Home Care and Hospice: Food Preparation and Safety

Topic: Food preparation and safety for the home care patient
Length: 20 minutes
Audience: Registered nurses, licensed vocational nurses, home health aides, other caregivers
Responsibility: Home health care dietitian
Goal: To familiarize personnel with safe food procurement, preparation, and storage
Objectives: Upon completion of this in-service, participants will be able to:

1. Identify three safety characteristics to look for when shopping for fresh and processed foods
2. Identify two food safety tips for foods that may cause food-borne illness
3. List appropriate temperatures at which to hold and store foods

Procedures: The dietitian will discuss:

1. Grocery shopping
   a. Meats, fish, poultry: Selecting fresh products, expiration dates
   b. Milk, dairy products: Pasteurization
   c. Fruits and vegetables: Selecting fresh products, unbroken skins
   d. Canned and frozen foods: Damaged products, thawing
   e. Eggs

2. Food preparation
   a. Shelf life: Expiration dates, labels
   b. Safe cooking methods: Temperatures, times
   c. Washing fruits and vegetables
   d. Cutting boards

3. Food storage
   a. Refrigerator and freezer: Time and temperature, labeling
   b. Dry and canned foods: Time, temperature, packaging

# In-service 9: Role of Nutrition in Palliative Care

Topic: Role of nutrition in palliative care
Length: 30 to 45 minutes
Audience: Registered nurses, licensed vocational nurses, home health aides
Responsibility: Dietitian
Goal: To familiarize health care providers and caretakers to the role of nutrition for the client at the end stage of HIV disease
Objectives: Upon completion of this in-service, participants will be able to:

1. Describe the role of food to the terminally ill client
2. Recognize clients who may benefit from nutrition intervention
3. List one intervention for each symptom discussed

Procedures: The dietitian will discuss:

1. Factors affecting the role of food in palliative and comfort care
   a. Emotional, physiological, sociological
   b. Religious, cultural
   c. Aversions, cravings

2. Referral criteria for dietitian
   a. Client request
   b. Symptom management
   c. Caretaker concerns about patient's inadequate intake

3. Symptom management
   a. Nausea, vomiting
   b. Xerostomia
   c. Malabsorption
   d. Constipation
   e. Diarrhea

# Appendix D
# Resources

**TABLE D-1** Food Programs Serving Meals to Clients With HIV and AIDS

| City | Name/Location/Telephone | Meals per Day | Comments |
|---|---|---|---|
| Baltimore | Moveable Feast<br>3401 Old York Rd<br>Baltimore, MD 21218<br>410/243-4604; fax: 410/243-3624 | >300 | Founded in 1989<br>Eligibility: Homebound persons with AIDS |
| Boston | Community Servings<br>1353 Dorchester Ave<br>Dorchester, MA 02122<br>617/287-1605; fax: 617/288-7297 | >250 | Founded in 1990<br>Eligibility: Homebound persons with AIDS and dependents |
| Chicago | Open Hand Chicago<br>1648 W Howard St<br>Chicago, IL 60626<br>773/665-1000; fax: 773/665-0044 | 1,500 | Founded in 1988<br>Eligibility: Persons with AIDS; dependents; caregivers |
| Cleveland | FACT: Facing the AIDS Challenge Together<br>2728 Euclid Ave, Suite 400<br>Cleveland, OH 44115<br>216/621-0766; fax: 216/622-7785 | 57 | Founded in 1993<br>Eligibility: Persons with AIDS |
| Columbus, Ohio | Project Open Hand Columbus<br>787 E Broad St<br>Columbus, OH 43205<br>614/221-5683; fax: 614/221-5633 | 100 | Founded in 1994<br>Eligibility: Symptomatic HIV-infected persons: homebound or limited in ability to cook or provide for own nutritional needs |
| Denver | Project Angel Heart<br>Denver Center for Living<br>915 E Ninth Ave<br>Denver, CO 80218<br>303/830-0202; fax: 303/830-1840 | >125 | Founded in 1991<br>Eligibility: Homebound persons with progressive chronic disease |

**TABLE D-1  Food Programs Serving Meals to Clients With HIV and AIDS (Continued)**

| City | Name/Location/Telephone | Meals per Day | Comments |
|---|---|---|---|
| Laguna Beach, Calif | Laguni Shanti<br>570 Glenneyre, Suite 100<br>Laguna Beach, CA 92651<br>714/494-1446; fax: 714/497-2496 | 75 | Founded in 1987<br>Eligibility: Homebound persons with HIV and AIDS |
| London | The Food Chain<br>25 Bertram St<br>London, N19 5DQ<br>England<br>44-171-272-2272; fax: 44-171-272-2273 | NA[a] | |
| Los Angeles | Project Angel Food<br>7474 Sunset Boulevard<br>Los Angeles, CA 90046<br>213/850-0877; fax: 213/650-2944 | >500 | Founded in 1989<br>Eligibility: Homebound persons with HIV and AIDS<br>Clients: 40% people of color |
| Miami | Food For Life Network<br>111 SW Third St<br>Miami, FL 33130<br>305/375-0400; fax: 305/375-8440 | >850 | Founded in 1987<br>Eligibility: Low-income persons with HIV and AIDS; homebound persons with AIDS |
| Minneapolis | Open Arms of Minnesota<br>500 Eighth Ave SE<br>Minneapolis, MN 55414<br>612/331-3640; fax: 612/331-3356 | 80 | Founded in 1987<br>Eligibility: HIV-positive persons |
| New Haven, Conn | Caring Cuisine AIDS Project<br>PO Box 636<br>New Haven, CT 06503<br>phone/fax: 203/624-0947 | 45 | Founded in 1987<br>Eligibility: Homebound persons with AIDS; dependents |
| New Orleans | Food for Friends<br>2533 Columbus St<br>New Orleans, LA 70119<br>504/944-6028; fax: 504/944-4441 | 400 | Founded in 1992<br>Eligibility: HIV- symptomatic persons; dependents |
| New York | God's Love We Deliver<br>166 Avenue of the Americas<br>New York, NY 10013<br>212/294-8100; fax: 212/294-8101 | 1,600 | Founded in 1985<br>Eligibility: Homebound persons with AIDS; dependents |
| Philadelphia | Metropolitan AIDS Neighborhood Nutrition Alliance (MANNA)<br>PO Box 30181<br>Philadelphia, PA 19103<br>215/496-2662; fax: 215/496-1349 | >100 | Founded in 1990<br>Eligibility: Homebound persons with AIDS; dependents<br>Clients: 25% women; 80% people of color |
| Portland, Ore | Ecumenical Ministries of Oregon/ HIV Center<br>3835 SW Kelly Ave<br>Portland, OR 97201<br>503/223-3444; fax: 503/223-3056 | 115 | Founded in 1990<br>Eligibility: HIV-positive status; tuberculosis (TB) clearance |
| Sacramento, Calif | Positive Gourmet Food Services<br>PO Box 160845<br>Sacramento, CA 95816<br>916/851-9850; fax: 916/851-9850 | — | Founded in 1994<br>Eligibility: Symptomatic persons with HIV or AIDS<br>Provide medical nutrition supplements |

## TABLE D-1 Food Programs Serving Meals to Clients With HIV and AIDS (Continued)

| City | Name/Location/Telephone | Meals per Day | Comments |
|---|---|---|---|
| St Louis | Food Outreach Inc<br>4579 Laclede Ave, Suite 309<br>St Louis, MO 63108<br>phone/fax: 314/367-4461 | >200 | Founded in 1988<br>Eligibility: HIV or AIDS |
| Salt Lake City | Utah AIDS Foundation<br>1408 South 1100 East<br>Salt Lake City, UT 84105<br>801/487-2323, fax: 801/486-3978 | 1 per person | Founded in 1985<br>Eligibility: Clients of agency; HIV-positive persons referred by physician |
| San Diego | Mama's Kitchen<br>2260 El Cajon Blvd, Suite 118<br>San Diego, CA 92104<br>619/589-1736; fax: 619/298-9830 | 500 | Founded in 1990<br>Eligibility: Homebound persons with AIDS |
| San Francisco area | Project Open Hand<br>730 Polk St, 3rd floor<br>San Francisco, CA 94109<br>415/558-0600; fax: 415/771-6571 | 1,800 | Founded in 1985<br>Eligibility: HIV-symptomatic persons |
| | Duboce StreetFood Bank<br>401 Duboce St<br>San Francisco, CA 94117 | | Clients: 40% people of color, 12% female |
| | Shattuck Avenue Food Bank<br>5720 Shattuck Ave<br>Oakland, CA 94609 | | Clients: 70% people of color, 20% female |
| San Rafael, Calif | Marin AIDS Project<br>1660 Second St<br>San Rafael, CA 94901-2702<br>415/457-2487; fax: 415/457-5687 | 35 | Founded in 1981<br>Eligibility: HIV-positive persons and those in financial need |
| Santa Fe, NM | Kitchen Angels<br>500 N Guadalupe, Suite 505<br>Santa Fe, NM 87501<br>505/471-7780; fax: 505/471-9632 | 60 | Founded in 1992<br>Eligibility: Homebound persons with HIV and AIDS under age 60 yr |
| Seattle | Chicken Soup Brigade<br>1002 E Seneca<br>Seattle, WA 98122<br>206/328-8979; fax: 206/328-0171 | 175 | Founded in 1983<br>Eligibility: HIV and AIDS |
| Washington, DC | Food and Friends<br>PO Box 70601<br>Washington, DC 20024<br>202/488-8278; fax: 202/863-1284 | >1,000 | Founded in 1988<br>Eligibility: Homebound persons with HIV and AIDS; dependents<br>Clients: 70% African-American; 20% female; 30% children and families |
| Vancouver, British Columbia, Canada | A Loving Spoonful<br>The Vancouver Meals Society<br>1300 Richards St, Suite 100<br>Vancouver, BC V6B 3G6<br>Canada | — | Delivers frozen meals weekly |

Source: Kraak V. Home-delivered meal programs for homebound people with HIV/AIDS. *J Am Diet Assoc*. 1995;95:476-481.
[a]NA indicates not available.

### TABLE D-2  Commercial Products

Abbott Laboratories
D-305 Building AP30-4E
1 Abbott Rd
Abbott Park, IL 60064
847/937-6100

Testoderm Patches
Alza Pharmaceuticals
950 Page Mill Rd
PO Box 10950
Palo Alto, CA 94303
415/494-5000

Megace®
Bristol-Myers Oncology
PO Box 4500
Princeton, NJ 08543
609/897-2000

BeneFit® Shake, Bars
HMR Inc
59 Temple Place, Suite 704
Boston, MA 02111
617/357-9876
800/467-6467

Lactaid™
Lactaid Hotline
PO Box 111
Pleasantville, NJ 08232
800/522-8243

ImmunAid®
McGaw Inc
2525 McGaw Ave
PO Box 19791
Irvine, CA 92714
714/660-2000
800/854-6851

HealthGain®
Metagenics Inc
971 Calle Negocio
San Clemente, CA 92673
714/366-0818
800/692-9400

NuBar®, SupplaCal®, other bar products
NCI Inc
5801 Ayala Ave
Irwindale, CA 91706
818/815-3393

Nutren®, NuBasics®, Reabilan®, Peptamen®, other liquid/bar supplements
Nestle
3 Pkwy N, Suite 500
PO Box 760
Deerfield, IL 60015
847/317-2800
800/422-2752

Impact®, Vivonex Plus®, others
Novartis
5320 W 23rd St
PO Box 370
Minneapolis, MN 55440
800/999-9978

Advera®, other supplements
Ross Laboratories
625 Cleveland Ave
Columbus, OH 43215
614/227-3333

Marinol®
Roxane Laboratories
PO Box 16532
Columbus, OH 43216
614/276-4000

Scandishake®, Ultrase® Pancreatic Enzymes, Mouth Kote®
Scandipharm Inc
22 Inverness Center Pkwy, Suite 200
Birmingham, AL 35242
205/991-8085

Serostim™ (rhGH)
Serono Laboratories Inc
100 Longwater Circle
Norwell, MA 02061
617/982-9000

Magnacal®
Sherwood Medical
1915 Olive St
St Louis, MO 63103
800/428-4400

## TABLE D-3 Professional Resources

**AIDS Education and Training Centers:**

New York/Virgin Islands AIDS ETC
Columbia University School of Public Health
600 W 168th St, 7th Floor
New York, NY 10032
Contact: Cheryl Healton, DrPH
212/305-3616; fax: 212/305-6832

Northwest AIDS ETC (Washington, Alaska, Montana, Idaho, Oregon)
University of Washington
1001 Broadway, Suite 217
Box 359932
Seattle, WA 98122
Contact: Ann Downer, MS
206/720-4250; fax: 206/720-4218

Great Lakes to Tennessee Valley AIDS ETC (Ohio, Michigan, Kentucky, Tennessee)
Wayne State University
2727 Second Ave, Room 142
Detroit, MI 48201
Contact: Ali M. Naqvi, PhD; Fredericka P. Shea, PhD, RN, FAAN
313/962-2000; fax: 313/962-4444

Pacific AIDS ETC (Nevada, Arizona, Hawaii, California)
University of California, San Francisco
5110 E Clinton Way, Suite 115
Fresno, CA 93727-2098
Contact: Michael Reyes, MD, MPH (western division)
209/252-2581; fax: 209/454-8012
Contact: Jerry Gates, PhD (southern division)
213/342-1846; fax: 213/342-2051

Southeast AIDS ETC (Alabama, Georgia, North Carolina, South Carolina)
Emory University
733 Gatewood Rd NE
Atlanta, GA 30322-4950
Contact: Ira Schwartz, MD
404/727-2929; fax: 404/727-4562

Delta Region AIDS ETC (Arkansas, Louisiana, Mississippi)
LSU Medical Center
136 Roman St, 3rd Floor
New Orleans, LA 70112
Contact: Jane Martin, MA, RN, FNP
504/568-3855; fax: 504/568-7893

Mountain Plains Regional AIDS ETC (North Dakota, South Dakota, Utah, Colorado, New Mexico, Nebraska, Kansas, Wyoming)
University of Colorado
4200 E Ninth Ave, Box A-096
Denver, CO 80262
Contact: Donna Anderson, PhD, MD
303/355-1301; fax: 303/355-1448

Midwest AIDS ETC (Illinois, Indiana, Iowa, Minnesota, Missouri, Wisconsin)
University of Illinois at Chicago
808 S Wood St (M/C 779)
Chicago, IL 60612-7303
Contact: Nathan L. Linsk, PhD; Barbara Schechtman, MPH
312/996-1373; fax: 312/413-4184

Mid-Atlantic AIDS ETC (Delaware, Maryland, Virginia, West Virginia, Washington, DC)
Virginia Commonwealth University
PO Box 980159
Richmond, VA 23298-0159
Contact: Lisa G. Kaplowitz
804/828-2447; fax: 804/828-1795

New England AIDS ETC (Connecticut, Maine, Massachusetts, New Hampshire, Rhode Island, Vermont)
320 Washington St, 3rd Floor
Brookline, MA 02146
Contact: Donna Gallagher, RN, MS, ANP
617/566-2283; fax: 617/566-2994

AIDS ETC for Texas and Oklahoma
The University of Texas
1200 Herman Pressler St
PO Box 20186
Houston, TX 77225
Contact: Richard Grimes, PhD
713/794-4075; fax: 713/792-5292

Pennsylvania AIDS ETC
University of Pittsburgh
Graduate School of Public Health
130 DeSoto St, Room A427
Pittsburgh, PA 15261
Contact: Linda Frank, PhD, MSN, RN
412/624-1895; fax: 412/624-4767

New Jersey AIDS ETC
University of Medicine and Dentistry of New Jersey
Center for Continuing Education
30 Bergen St, ADMC #710
Newark, NJ 07107-3000
Contact: Debra Bartelli, MA, MPH
201/982-3690; fax: 201/982-7128

Florida AIDS ETC
University of Miami Department of Family Medicine
South Shore Hospital
600 Alton Rd, Suite 502
Miami Beach, FL 33139
Contact: Cynthia Carmichael, MD
305/531-1224, ext 3549; fax: 305/532-9604

## TABLE D-3 Professional Resources (Continued)

**AIDS Education and Training Centers: (Continued)**
Puerto Rico AIDS ETC
University of Puerto Rico Medical Sciences Campus
GPO 36-5067, Room A-956
San Juan, Puerto Rico 00936-5067
Contact: Daisy M. Gely, MPHE
809/759-6528; fax: 809/764-2470
Contact: Angel Bravo, MPH
809/756-7931; fax: 809/764-4951

American Foundation for AIDS Research (AmFAR)
AIDS/HIV Treatment Directory
212/682-7440

AIDS Project Los Angeles (APLA)
1313 N Vine St
Los Angeles, CA 90028
213/993-1611

AIDS Targeted Information (ATIN)
800/392-6327

AIDS Drug Assistance Program (ADAP)
800/542-2437

AIDS Medications in Development
Pharmaceutical Manufacturers Association
Communication Division
1100 15th St NW
Washington, DC 20005
202/835-3400

American Academy of Pediatrics (AAP)
141 Northwest Point Blvd
Elk Grove Village, IL 60009
800/433-9016

American Dietetic Association (ADA)
216 W Jackson Blvd
Chicago, IL 60606
800/877-1600
Nutrition hot line: National Center for Nutrition and Dietetics
800/366-1655

American Medical Association (AMA)
515 N State St
Chicago, IL 60610
312/464-5000

American Public Health Association (APHA)
Food and Nutrition Section
1015 15th St NW
Washington, DC 20005
202/789-5600

American Society of Health-System Pharmacists
(publishes American Hospital Formulary Service drug information yearly)
7272 Wisconsin Ave
Bethesda, MD 20814
301/657-4383

American Society for Parenteral and Enteral Nutrition (ASPEN)
8605 Cameron St, Suite 500
Silver Spring, MD 20910
301/587-6315

Association of Nurses in AIDS Care
11250 Roger Bacon Dr, Suite 8
Reston, VA 22090
800/260-6780

Bulletin of Experimental Treatments for AIDS (BETA)
San Francisco AIDS Foundation
25 Van Ness Ave, Suite 600
San Francisco, CA 94102
415/864-5855, ext 2031
800/959-1059

Centers for Disease Control and Prevention (CDC)
Fax Line Information: 404/332-4565
Division of Nutrition
1600 Clifton Rd NE, MS K-24
Atlanta, GA 30333
404/488-5134

Food and Drug Administration (FDA)
Office of Consumer Affairs
5600 Fishers Ln, HFE-88
Rockville, MD 20857
301/443-3170

Gay Men's Health Crisis
129 W 20th St
New York, NY 10011
212/337-1950

National Association for People With AIDS
1413 K St NW
Washington, DC 20005
202/898-0414
Fax Line Information: 202/789-2222

National AIDS Clearinghouse
Fax Line Information: 800/458-5231

National AIDS Hot Line
800/342-2437 (English)
800/344-7432 (Spanish)

National Cancer Institute
Bldg 31, 10A-24
9000 Rockville Pike
Bethesda, MD 20892
800/422-6237

National Hospice Organization
1901 North Moore St, Suite 901
Arlington, VA 22209
703/253-5900

**TABLE D-3　Professional Resources (Continued)**

Nutritionists in AIDS Care
PO Box 760
Lennox Hill Station
New York, NY 10021
212/439-8073

Oley Foundation
Albany Medical Center
214 Hun Memorial
Albany, NY 12208
518/262-5079

Philadelphia FIGHT
201 N Broad St, 6th Floor
Philadelphia, PA 19107
215/557-8265

Project Inform
1965 Market St, Suite 220
San Francisco, CA 94103
415/558-8669
800/822-7422

Test Positive Aware (TPA) Network
1258 W Belmont Ave
Chicago, IL 60657
773/404-8726

AIDS Treatment News
PO Box 411256
San Francisco, CA 94141
415/255-0588

Women and AIDS Resource Network (WARN)
PO Box 020525
Brooklyn, NY 11202
718/596-6007

**For a comprehensive listing of Canadian resources, contact:**

Canadian AIDS Society
100 Sparks St, Suite 400
Ottawa, Ontario K1P 5B7
Canada
613/230-3580; fax: 613/563-4998

National AIDS Clearinghouse (NAC)
1565 Carling Ave, Suite 400
Ottawa, Ontario K1Z 8R1
Canada
613/725-3434

**In England, contact:**

FACTS
23-25 Weston Park
Crouch End, London N8 9SY
England
081-348 9195

## TABLE D-4  Buyer's Clubs

Buyer's clubs are collective organizations that buy and distribute experimental medications, vitamins and minerals, supplements, and drugs approved in other countries. These groups often collect information on these treatments and many monitor effects that their users report.

| City | Club | Telephone |
|---|---|---|
| Atlanta | AIDS Treatment Initiatives | 404/874-4845 |
| Boston | PWA Coalition Boston | 617/266-6422 |
|  | Boston Buyer's Club | 800/435-5586 |
|  |  | 617/266-2223 |
| Capitola, CA | Embrace Life | 800/448-1170 |
| Chicago | Surviving With AIDS Naturally | 312/561-2800 |
| Dallas | DBC Alternatives | 214/528-4460 |
| Denver | Colorado Health Action Project | 303/837-8214 |
|  | Denver Buyer's Club | 303/329-9379 |
| Fort Lauderdale, Fla | Health Link | 305/565-8284 |
|  | Wholesale Health | 954/764-1587 |
| Houston | Prince Street Market | 713/520-5288 |
| New York City | DAAIR | 212/689-8140 |
|  | PWA Health Group | 212/255-0520 |
|  | Direct AIDS Alternative Information Resources | 212/725-6994 |
| Phoenix | Being Alive Buyer's Club | 602/265-2437 |
|  | Phoenix Body Positive | 602/955-4673 |
| San Francisco | Healing Alternatives Foundation | 800/219-2233 |
|  |  | 415/626-4053 |
| Sarasota, Fla | AIDS Manasota | 941/954-6011 |
| Tucson, Ariz | PACT for Life Buyer's Club | 520/770-1710 |
| Washington, DC | Carl Vogel Foundation | 202/638-0750 |

## TABLE D-5  Current Clinical Trials

CenterWatch Inc Publication Company
581 Boylston St
Boston, MA 02116
617/247-2327; Fax: 617/247-2535
E-mail: cntrwatch@aol.com

## TABLE D-6  Suggested Resources for HIV Case Managers

**WWW and the Internet**

*AIDS Treatment News*
Web site: http://www.aidsnews.org

AIDSLINE, AIDS TRIALS, AIDS DRUGS
A Guide to the National Library of Medicine's AIDS Databases
Web site: http://www.med.harvard.edu/countway/aidsdb.html

CDC Daily Information
Web site: http://www.cdc.gov

*Journal of the American Medical Association* (HIV and AIDS):
Web site: http://www.ama-assn.org/special/hiv/hivhome.html

National Library of Medicine
Web site: http.nlm.nih.gov/aidspubl.html

Project Inform
Web site: http://www.projinf.org

**Hot Lines (Pacific Standard Time)**

HIV Telephone Consult for CCMs (CPAT)
800/933-3413

Physician's Clinical Support
310/443-4231

**Special Resources**

Being Alive
213/667-3262

Positively Aware
312/404-8726

WO.R.L.D. (Women Organized to Respond to Life-threatening Diseases)
510/658-6930

*The Journal of Care Management* (journal of CMSA, Case Management Society of America)
203/454-2300

CMSA
501/225-2229

POZ
349 W 12th St
New York, NY 10014
800/973-2376; fax: 212/675-8505
E-mail: Pozmag@aol.com

**Miscellaneous**

*Applying Medical Case Management: AIDS*
Thorn, 1990
805/944-3312

Activist organizations, buyer's clubs, and Persons With AIDS coalitions
415/861-7505

# Index

## A

Acquired immunodeficiency syndrome. *See* AIDS
Activities of daily living (ADL), 109
Acute retroviral syndrome (ARS), 21, 113
Aerobic exercise, 38
Africa, 1, 2, 6
AIDS
  cause of death, 13
  compared to plague, 1
  defining diseases, 4
  definitions, 3-6, 4, 113
  history of, 2-3
  laboratory tests for, 6
  nutrition and. *See* Nutrition therapy
  opportunistic infections, 10-12, 116
  polls, 1
  statistics, 1, 8-9, 58
AIDS-related complex (ARC), 6, 113
Albumin, 28, 72
Alternative therapies, 56-57, 113
American Medical Association, 56
Anemia, 30
Anorexia, 48-49
Anthropometric measurements, 24-28, 138, 142. *See also specific types*
Antibacterial medications, 32
Antibodies, 113
Antifungal medications, 32
Antigen, 113
Antiprotozoal medications, 32-33
Antiretroviral drugs. *See* Protease inhibitors
Antiviral medications, 33
Appetite stimulation, 49
Aspiration, 79
Australia, 2
AZT. *See* Zidovudine

## B

Barrett, S, 56
Beal, JE, 49
Behavioral outcomes, 110-111
Biochemical values, 28-33
Bioelectrical impedance analysis (BIA), 22, 27-28
  body composition, 143
  machines, 28
  reports, 142-145
Blesi, B, 108, 109
Blood-borne disease, 114
Body cell mass (BCM), 25, 27
Body mass index (BMI), 25, 137
Breast-feeding. *See* Lactation
Bubonic plague, 1
Buyer's clubs, 173

## C

Canada, 2
Candidiasis, 10, 114
Case managers, 174
CD4 cell levels, 2, 6-7, 21, 40, 53, 104
CD8 cell levels, 6-7
Centers for Disease Control and Prevention (CDC), 4, 21, 114
Cervical cancer, 10
Chandra, RK, 13-14
Chemokines, 3
Chicken Brigade (Seattle), 108-109
Clinical outcomes, 110
Clinical trials, 97, 117
Clinics, 97-99, 101
Coccidioidomycosis, 10
Coccidiosis, 11
Cofactor, 114
Community programs, 106-109
Connor, EM, 60
Constipation, 53, 79
Counseling, 22, 44, 57-58, 97-99, 107
  centers for AIDS education, 170-172
  health professionals, 146-165
  in-service for enteral support, 155-161
  in-service for home care, 163-164
  in-service for hospice care, 163-164
  in-service for immunology, 146-150
  in-service for nutrition assessment,

151-153
    in-service for nutrition therapy, 146-165
    in-service for nutritional products, 154
    in-service for palliative care, 165
Cryptococcal meningitis, 10
Cryptosporidiosis, 10, 114
*Cryptosporidium*, 14, 35
Cytokine, 114
Cytomegalovirus (CMV), 10, 114

**D**
Dehydration, 53
Dementia, 10
Dextrose, 85
Diarrhea, 10, 52-53, 79
Diet, 47-48, 107-108. *See also* Food groups
    consistency of food, 96
    content of food, 96
Dietitian. *See also specific topics*
    employment in home health, 103
    teamwork and, 90, 161
Discharge, 98-99
Disinfectant, 114
Dronabinol, 49
Drug-nutrient interactions, 30-33
Dysgeusia, 50

**E**
Electrolytes, 85-86
Energy requirements, 68, 72
Enteral support, 73-80, 155-161
    biochemical alterations, 69-71
    bolus feedings, 75
    complications, 78-79
    conditions that justify, 75
    cyclic feedings, 75
    decision tree, 74
    efficacy, 78
    feeding indications, 75
    feeding routes, 75
    feeding tubes, 78
    formulas, 73-75, 157
    infusion options, 75-76
    management, 79-80
    monitoring, 79-80, 81, 82, 158
    product sampling, 76-77
Enzyme-linked immunosorbent assay (ELISA), 6, 114
Europe, 2
Exercise, 37-38
Extracellular mass (ECM), 27
Extracellular tissue (ECT), 27

**F**
Fenton, M, 107, 109
Fluid requirements, 67-68
Food and Drug Administration, 114
Food-borne infection, 14
Food choice. *See* Diet
Food groups, 145
Food preparation, 164
Food programs, 166-168
Food safety, 44-47, 108-109, 164
Food stamps, 105, 107
Friendly Hills Health Care Network, 106
Functional outcomes, 110
Fungus, 114

**G**
Gastrointestinal problems, 15, 33-34, 103, 108
Gibson, RS, 38
God's Love We Deliver (GLWD), 104-105, 107-108, 167
Groceries-to-Go, 109

**H**
Hairy leukoplakia, 10
Hand-grip dynamometry, 38, 145
Health care service
    cost, 104
    race and, 104
    use of by people with HIV, 104-105
Health care settings, 93-111
    clinics, 97-99, 101
    home, 99-103, 163-164
    hospices, 109-110, 115, 163-164
    hospital, 93-97, 162
    inpatient setting, 93-97, 162
Height measurement, 24, 137
Hemophilia, 114
Hepatitis B, 114
Herpes, 11, 115
Histoplasmosis, 11
HIV
    clinical categories, 22-24
    clinical manifestations, 9-13
    definitions, 3-6, 115
    drug intervention, 5
    life cycle, 5
    mother-to-child transmission, 60-61, 117-118
    opportunistic infections, 10-12, 116
    pathophysiological process, 6-7
    stages, 21-24
    strains, 6
    transmission, 8, 60-61, 117-118
Home care, 99-103, 163-164
Hospices, 109-110, 115, 163-164
Hospital care, 93-97, 162
Hot lines, 174
Human immunodeficiency virus. *See* HIV
Human papillomavirus, 11
Human T-cell lymphotropic virus, type III, 115
Hypophosphatemia, 86

**I**
ICD-9 codes, 29
Ideal body weight (IBW), 25, 68
Immune modulator medications, 33
Immunoglobulin, 115
Immunology, 146-150
In-services. *See* Counseling
Incidence, 115
Incubation, 115
Indinavir, 33
Indinavir sulfate, 3
Infection, 10-12, 115
Infectious disease, 115
Interferons, 115
Interleukin-2, 115
International Conference on AIDS, 3
Internet, 174
Intervention. *See* Nutrition therapy

**J**
Jain, VK, 13-14
Johnson, M, 8
Joint Commission on Accreditation of Healthcare Organizations (JCAHO), 94, 95, 102-103, 109, 111

**K**
Kaposi sarcoma, 3, 11, 115
Karnofsky Scale, 21, 136
Kruse, LM, 105, 109

**L**
Laboratory tests for AIDS, 6
Laboratory values, 28-29
Lactation, 58-59, 60
    breast-feeding decisions, 61
Lean body mass (LBM), 21, 25, 38
Lentivirus, 115

Lesion, 115
Lipids, 85
Lymph glands, 116
Lymphadenopathy-associated virus (LAV), 116
Lymphocytes, 116
Lymphoma, 11, 116

## M

Macrophage, 116
Magestrol acetate, 48
Magnesium, 90
Malnutrition, 13-15. *See also* Nutrition therapy
  assessment, 29
  cachexia-related wasting, 66
  causes of, 43
  protein-energy manutrition, 24, 150
  signs of, 36-37
  starvation-related, 66
Managed care, 105-106
Meals
  congregate, 107
  home-delivered, 104, 107
  programs, 166-168
Medicaid, 105, 116
Medical history, 37, 44
Medical nutrition therapy protocol for HIV/AIDS, 22, 44, 110-111, 121-135
Medicare, 116
Medications. *See also specific types*
  combination drug therapy, 30
  interactions, 30-33
  side effects, 30-33
Megesterol acetate, 30
Meningitis, 116
Micronutrient supplements, 73, 85, 86. *See also* Minerals; Vitamins
Midarm circumference (MAC), 26, 140-142
Midarm muscle circumference, 26-27, 140-141
Minerals, 53-54, 57, 73
  effects on immune functions, 149
  for parenteral support, 85-87, 90
  during pregnancy, 59
  trace elements, 86-87
Monocyte, 116
Mouth pain, 49-50
Mucous membrane, 116
Multicenter AIDS Cohort Study (MACS), 104
*Mycobacterium avium* complex (MAC), 11, 35, 116

## N

National Institute of Allergy and Infectious Disease (NIAID), 116
National Institutes of Health (NIH), 116
Nausea, 49, 79
Nelfinavir mesylate, 3
Neutropenia, 116
New Zealand, 2
Nurse, teamwork and, 161
Nutrients. *See also* Minerals; *specific types*; Vitamins
  immune system and, 149-150
Nutrition education. *See* Counseling
Nutrition monitoring, 18, 45
  in hospitals, 94-95
Nutrition screening, 18-21, 95, 102, 163
Nutrition supplements, 51, 54-56. *See also* Minerals; Vitamins
Nutrition therapy, 13-15, 110. *See also* Counseling; Enteral support; Malnutrition; Parenteral support
  assessment, 24, 67, 93-111, 151-153
  clinical categories and, 22-24
  in clinics, 97-99, 101
  community programs, 106-109
  drug-nutrient interactions, 30-33
  energy requirements, 68, 72
  flow sheet, 102
  fluid requirements, 67-68
  goals for, 65-67
  home care, 99-103
  in hospices, 109-110
  in hospitals, 93-97
  ICD-9 codes for, 29
  immunology and, 146-150
  individualized, 44, 67, 97
  laboratory tests, 19
  micronutrient supplements, 73
  nutrient intake, 35, 37, 38
  oral. *See* Oral nutrition intervention
  outcomes, 38-40, 67, 109-110
  prenatal care, 59-60
  protein, 47, 72
  referrals, 19, 21, 100

## O

Open Hand (Atlanta), 109

Opportunistic infections, 10-12, 116
Oral nutrition intervention, 43-60
Orphan drug, 116
Outpatients, 97-99

## P

p24 antigen, 116
Palliative care, 165
Parenteral support, 80-91, 159-163
  biochemical alterations, 69-71
  complications, 87-88
  conditions that justify, 75
  decision tree, 74
  efficacy, 90
  infection control, 88
  management, 88-90
  monitoring, 82, 88-90
  role of dietitian in, 90
  routes, 83, 84
  solutions, 83-85
  team approach, 90
PCP. *See Pneumocystis carinii* pneumonia
Pelvic inflammatory disease, 12
Perinatal transmission, 60-61, 117
Peripheral neuropathy, 12
Persistent generalized lymphadenopathy (PGL), 117
Pharmacist, 161
Phase angles, 27
Physical therapist, teamwork and, 161
Physician, teamwork and, 161
Plasma albumin, 28
*Pneumocystis carinii* pneumonia, 2, 3, 9, 12, 35, 94, 117
Polymerase chain reaction (PCR), 117
Prealbumin transferrin, 28
Pregnancy, 44, 58-60
  mother-to-child transmission of HIV, 60-61, 117
  weight gain, 60
Prenatal care, 59-60
Prevalence, 117
Preventive nutrition care, 105
Products
  commercial, 169
  for enteral support, 77-78
  medical nutritional, 154
Progressive multifocal leukoencephalopathy, 12
Progressive resistance training, 37-38
Project Open Hand (San

Francisco), 108, 168
Prophylaxis, 117
Prospective cohort, 117
Prospective study, 117
Protease inhibitors, 2, 3, 30, 31-32, 117
Protein, 47, 72
Protein-energy manutrition, 24, 150
Provirus, 117

**R**

Recommended Daily Allowances (RDA), 47, 73
"Refeeding syndrome," 86
Resistance exercise, 37
Resources, professional, 170-172, 174
Respite care, 117
Retinol-binding protein, 28-29
Retrovirus, 118
Reverse transcriptase, 7, 118
Risk behaviors, 8, 118
Risk group, 118
Ritonavir, 3
Ryan White Comprehensive AIDS Resources Emergency Act, 105

**S**

Safer sex, 118
Salmonellosis, 12
Saquinavir, 30
Saquinavir mesylate, 3
*Science*, 3, 7
Sensitivity, 118
Seroconversion, 6, 118
Seropositive, 118
Serum albumin, 28
Shingles, 118
Silverman, E, 106
Skinfold measurements. *See* Triceps skinfold
Smallpox, 1
Social history, 37
Specificity, 118
Swallowing, 49-50

**T**

T cells, 2, 118. *See also* CD4 cell levels
Tang, AM, 53
Taste alterations, 50
Tat gene, 118
Taxoplasmosis, 12
Team approach, 90, 94, 161
Total parenteral support (TPN), 83. *See also* Parenteral support
Toxoplasmosis, 118
Trace elements, 86-87
Transcriptase inhibitors, 31
Triceps skinfold (TSF), 22, 26-27, 94, 138-139, 142
  for black adults, 139
  procedures, 142
  for white adults, 138
Triglyceride, 85
Tuberculosis, 9, 12, 118

**U**

Upper arm muscle area (UAMA), 26-27
US Food and Drug Administration (FDA), 3
Usual body weight (UBW), 25

**V**

Vaccine, 118
Van Roenn, JH, 48
Vector, 118
Vegetarians, 44
Vertical transmission, 60, 118
Viral load, 119
testing, 3, 7-8
Virus, 119
Visiting Nurse Association and Hospice (San Francisco), 100
Visiting Nurse Service (New York), 100
Vitamins, 53-54, 73
  B-12, 30
  C, 57
  during pregnancy, 59
  E, 57
  effects on immune function, 149-150
  for parenteral support, 85-87
Vomiting, 49

**W**

Walter Reed Staging Classification, 21, 136
Wasting syndrome, 119. *See also* Weight loss
Water systems, 14
Weight loss, 6, 12, 24-26, 38-30, 66
Weight measurement, 24-26, 137
Western blot test, 6, 119
White, R, 8
White blood cell, 119
WIC programs, 107

**X**

Xerostomia, 51

**Y**

Yale-New Haven Hospital Nutritional Classification and Assessment Program, 94

**Z**

Zidovudine, 2, 30, 60